ADDITIONAL PRAISE FOR

Yoga for Emotional Balance

"Bo Forbes brilliantly illuminates the fa
depressed or anxious as well as your mind. 1
the habitual postures and movements of
can be corrected through the practices she describes, leading to
dramatically improved mood states. Highly recommended!"

—ANDREW WEIL, MD

"*Yoga for Emotional Balance* reveals, with humor and delightful
examples, the enormous potential of restorative yoga for creating a
rich and bright emotional world."

— RICHARD FREEMAN, author of *The Mirror of Yoga*

"I am very pleased to give my highest recommendation to *Yoga
for Emotional Balance*. What shines through most clearly on every
page is Bo Forbes' voice—down-to-earth, knowledgeable, and above
all—compassionate."

— LESLIE KAMINOFF, co-author of *Yoga Anatomy*

"*Yoga for Emotional Balance* unpacks the complexity of the mind-
body relationship in an accessible and practical way, illustrating the
power of yoga to create physiological and psych-emotional change.
Bo Forbes' book is full of stories, processes, and insight—leaving
the reader with a roadmap to emotional balance."

— GARY KRAFTSOW, author of *Yoga for Wellness*

"Bo Forbes' voice throughout this book is consistently inviting
and gracious, deeply and confidently knowledgeable. Readers will
feel hopeful as soon as they start to read this book, even before
beginning to practice the remarkably accessible exercises."

—SYLVIA BOORSTEIN, author of *Happiness Is an Inside Job*

"This is precisely this kind of clear, accessible instruction that will catalyze both the lay and scientific communities to take these practices more seriously and explore their impact."
—RICHARD J. DAVIDSON, professor of Psychology and Psychiatry, and director of The Center for Investigating Healthy Minds, University of Wisconsin–Madison

"Bo Forbes has shown us a path to emotional balance that is located right here inside our bodies! I noticed more trust in my inner capacity for healing after reading this book."
—DAVID RICHO PhD, author of *When the Past Is Present*

"After reading Bo Forbes' book, I was eager to practice deep relaxation immediately! Highly recommended for all levels of yoga students."
—JUDITH HANSON LASATER, PhD, PT, author of *Yogabody: Anatomy, Kinesiology, and Asana*

"Written with insight, elegance, and wit, this book is a must-read for yoga teachers, therapists, students, laypeople, and anyone looking for alternatives to modern methods of healing."
—EDWIN BRYANT, professor of Hindu Religion and Philosophy, Rutgers University

Yoga for Emotional Balance

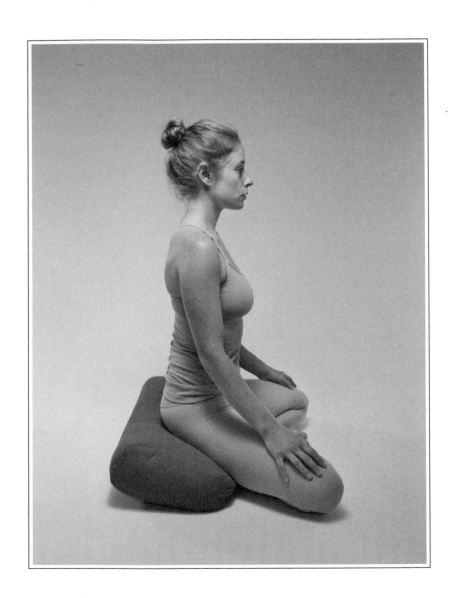

YOGA *for* Emotional Balance

Simple Practices to Help Relieve Anxiety and Depression

Bo Forbes, PsyD

Photographs by
Thibaut Fagonde

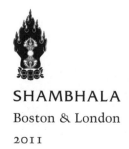

SHAMBHALA
Boston & London
2011

Shambhala Publications, Inc.
Horticultural Hall
300 Massachusetts Avenue
Boston, Massachusetts 02115
www.shambhala.com

9 8 7 6 5 4 3 2 1

FIRST EDITION
Designed by Steve Dyer
Printed in the United States of America

⊗ This edition is printed on acid-free paper that meets the
American National Standards Institute z39.48 Standard.
♻ This book was printed on 30% postconsumer recycled
paper. For more information, please visit www.shambhala.com.
Distributed in the United States by Random House, Inc.,
and in Canada by Random House of Canada Ltd

Library of Congress Cataloging-in-Publication Data
Forbes, Bo.
Yoga for emotional balance: simple practices to help relieve anxiety
and depression / Bo Forbes. — 1st ed.
p.   cm.
Includes bibliographical references.
ISBN 978-1-59030-760-1 (pbk.: alk. paper)
1. Yoga—Therapeutic use. 2. Anxiety. 3. Depression, Mental.
I. Title.
RA781.7.F67 2011
613.7'046—dc22
2010023011

To all my past, present, and future students,
who are also my wise and generous teachers.

Suffering is the breaking of the shell that
Encloses our understanding.

— Kahlil Gibran

CONTENTS

PREFACE

My journey to understanding yoga's connection with emotional balance has been a lifelong one. I grew up with a natural desire to heal others, and the subject of emotional health and healing captivated my attention. For my eighteenth birthday, my father gave me a copy of *Light on Yoga* by B. K. S. Iyengar. I set the book aside, and it would be another ten years before I cracked it open. I was on another path, one with a single-pointed focus on psychology. One year later, at the University of Chicago, I took graduate classes in social work and dove into the world of the mind and emotions. My peers and I examined our family histories and studied the emotional climate of college life around us. What *is* emotional health? I wondered. Why do some people have it without seeming to try, while others seek it fruitlessly all their lives? My investigations showed me that a difficult childhood doesn't necessarily condemn us to future pain and suffering. Some people find emotional well-being despite childhood abuse; others can fall apart even with family stability on their side. What qualities make up emotional balance, I wanted to know, and how can I help people develop them? I earned a doctorate in clinical psychology and, in my postgraduate work, continued to investigate the mysteries of emotional health.

For the first five years, I found fulfillment in my psychotherapy practice. My clients got better: they reported a drop in anxiety, fewer instances of deep depression, and less conflict in their primary relationships. And yet, I couldn't shake the feeling that psychotherapy was missing something. To complement my clinical practice, I investigated body-centered and spiritual approaches to emotional health. I tried everything from acupuncture to hands-on healing to see if they held promise for my clients.

I'd exercised most of my life and felt its stress-relieving benefits. But nothing, it turns out, spoke to me as powerfully as the well-being I felt after my first yoga class. The teacher, a ninety-seven-year-old woman on the South Side of Chicago named Becky Love (she drove a black Cadillac whose license plate read "YOGA"), had *exuberance*. She delighted in both movement and stillness. She really *felt* her body. She called us "Dear Ones" and exulted when one of her students went deeper into a pose ("*Look* at Tanya!" she'd exclaim. Or, "Look at *Edward!*"). When class ended, she offered us a sample of whatever wild new superfood she'd brought that day (kombucha mushroom tea or spirulina powder, long before they were in vogue) and then motored off to Whole Foods for brunch. Becky radiated well-being; it was contagious. But my interest went beyond that. Yoga calmed my mind. It felt like a deeper way of coming into my body than exercise. It also gave me a strong sense of inner connection. If yoga could make *me* feel this good, I wondered, what might it do for people with anxiety and depression? Could yoga—with its influence on mind, body, *and* spirit—be the missing piece I'd sought all this time?

At first, yoga seemed impossible to reconcile with psychotherapy. The main obstacle in my path was that in the early 1990s, when I began my postdoctoral employment, the body was forbidden territory for most psychologists. But this prohibition couldn't stand up to my personal experience of yoga's emotional benefits. I began to study yoga alongside my clinical work, and became the butt of many tiresome "granola" and "incense-burning" jokes among the board members at my group psychotherapy practice. At the time, it seemed necessary to choose one career over the other, and I thought about leaving psychotherapy to train as a yoga teacher.

The more I practiced yoga, however, the more I realized that psychotherapy and yoga are a natural fit. Psychotherapy features a rich collaborative relationship between client and therapist, and is eloquent in addressing the mind and emotions. Yoga is fluent in the language of the physical body, yet also affects the mind. Therapy (which comes from the Greek *therapeia*, "to heal") is integrative and truly healing when it involves the mind *and* body.

The next several years of clinical work convinced me that the body holds an essential key to healing anxiety and depression. It might even play an integral role in closing the gap between intellectual insight—the understanding of *why* we sometimes make destructive choices—and lasting change, the practice of *how* to make healthier ones. When we don't involve the body in treatment, we keep psychotherapy mind-based, and leave out an important part of the healing process.

Many people tell me excitedly how much yoga helps them, not just physically but emotionally. Some are wedded to fast-paced, physically demanding classes such as Ashtanga or Vinyasa Yoga. Others swear by "hot yoga" practices like Bikram or Power Yoga. Still others are devoted to Iyengar Yoga or to slower forms of physical practice. No matter the style of yoga, people report feeling mentally calmer, more physically energized, and happier after practicing. They also say that when they don't practice yoga for a while, their emotional challenges resume in full force. Even a regular yoga class has a healing impact, so I wondered what would happen if I chose the most therapeutic elements of yoga and used them with deliberate intention to heal emotional issues such as anxiety and depression.

Despite the fears of family and friends that I was "throwing away my doctorate," I incorporated yoga into my psychotherapy practice. For several years, I worked with clients referred by local alternative health centers who were more open to yoga-influenced psychotherapy. I watched clients carefully to see which elements of yoga were most helpful for anxiety, depression, insomnia, and other issues. I noted how certain practices increased energy for people with depression, and how others grounded and calmed individuals with anxiety. The results were hard to dismiss: people got better more fully and rapidly when I integrated yoga postures and breathing exercises into psychotherapy than they did with traditional psychotherapy alone. Despite these encouraging results, I remained a "closet yogi" in the world of psychology, where yoga was considered a fringe activity. And in the yoga world, where psychology was extraneous and a little uncool, I rarely told anyone what I did for a living.

During my first five years of teaching yoga, my practice and teaching styles centered on the physically active Vinyasa and alignment-based Iyengar Yoga practices until I made a sudden discovery. I began to teach Restorative Yoga, a restful, rejuvenative "yogic relaxation" class directly after my Vinyasa class. The week following each class, my longtime students who'd stayed for Restorative Yoga would tell me excitedly that they'd suddenly slept better, had less anxiety, or felt more physically and emotionally energized than before. Some even experienced improvements in physical illness or pain levels. At first, I found it hard to believe; with such powerful active practices at our fingertips, why would a seemingly "passive" relaxation class produce such dramatic results in us? But it happened month after month and year after year: Restorative Yoga and breathing exercises, the techniques featured in this book, were the most effective of all styles of yoga.

The yoga community in the West, myself included, has become so engrossed in the beauty and power of active practices and difficult postures that we can overlook the therapeutic benefits of "quieter" yoga. We've created a paradigm of yoga that entails continual movement without much space for intentioned reflection. People who prefer a physically challenging practice may find this hard to accept: with as little as fifteen to thirty minutes of twice-weekly breathing exercises and Restorative Yoga, people's thinking can become less emotionally reactive. They grow more able to tolerate challenging emotions. They become less anxious, less depressed. They begin to develop the qualities and skills that we psychotherapists work so hard to help instill. I've seen this time after time in my clients.

I've also noticed something else. When Restorative Yoga and simple breathing exercises helped people become more balanced, sometimes they'd try to describe their improvement to me or "analyze" why the practice worked so well. Inevitably, the analysis brought them back into their minds, where anxiety and depression were churning. Jeremy,[1] a young advertising executive, wanted to mentally process every improvement he experienced in his sessions. The more he'd leap up from his mat to talk about the calmness in his mind and the lightness or freedom in his body, the more that new, hard-to-describe feeling receded like a mirage in the desert. In order to process the change, Jeremy had to abandon his direct experience of it. Yet when he simply stayed present in his body, he could surrender and truly experience the positive changes happening inside him. When Jeremy finally "got it," he was very excited. "One of these sessions," he said, "is like eight months of psychotherapy."

As a psychotherapist, I didn't expect to see the positive results increase so significantly when I took much of the psychotherapy—the verbal processing—out of the session. But they did. Observing this, I began to use less verbal processing and more yoga in my clinical practice. This made an immediate and noticeable difference to my clients: it improved their mood, increased their self-compassion, and gave them a stronger sense of connection with others. When I say this at national yoga workshops, the psychotherapists in the audience almost always agree: you don't need to understand or even process your thoughts or emotions in order to experience dramatic shifts in mood, behavior, and well-being.

Think for a moment: How many times have you known what your issues are, yet not been able to change them? In other words, the talking part of the session is not the only, or perhaps not even the primary, key to change. *Conceptual insight is not required for change; in some cases it actually interferes with it.* By working in a body-based realm, we can bypass this mental interference. We can *feel* rather than *think* the emotional experiences that heal us.

This discovery rocked my professional world. To be honest, I grieved over it almost as much as I celebrated it. For many psychotherapists, the ability to process is an almost-sacred gift. Language is the medium through which we share that gift with our clients. We spend years (and considerable resources) refining the art of listening, interpreting, and reflecting back what our clients tell us. Although the art of mindful listening is important, *words* breathe this art to life. Yet despite my mixed feelings about it, therapy consistently yielded better results when clients *practiced* more than they *processed.*

Time passed, and notwithstanding my own early skepticism and that of my colleagues, psychiatrists and health centers began to send me a steady stream of patients with anxiety, depression, and chronic pain. One psychiatrist confided that this "yoga therapy stuff" was helping him take his client where he'd wanted her to go for many years.

Over the last two decades, my work as a psychologist has taken me to psychiatric hospitals and outpatient clinics, group practice and private practice. My work as a yoga teacher and yoga therapist has brought me to athletic stadiums, yoga studios, retreat centers, national conferences, and living rooms. I've treated the "worried well," people with moderate anxiety and depression, and individuals in severe emotional distress. Out of thirty years' combined experience in practicing psychotherapy and teaching yoga, I've synthesized the healing philosophies and practices of yoga and psychology into a unique practice that I call "Integrative Yoga Therapeutics" because it treats the mind and body simultaneously. It also treats that ineffable part of us that exists beyond the mind and body: our spirit, or vital essence.

A person with mild to moderate anxiety or depression can practice the exercises outlined in this book *as a companion* to traditional psychotherapy or medication and see dramatic improvement. And while this may sound radical, the benefits can extend even further. I don't mean to minimize the impact of psychotherapy or medication. They are often essential to survival and a positive quality of life. But when it's not a matter of life, death, or significant disability, regular practice of therapeutic yoga enables many people (with a doctor's and therapist's supervision) to lower and sometimes discontinue medication. Let me emphasize: this doesn't mean that you need to give up psychotherapy or medication in order to practice yoga. Nor do you have to give up the active style of yoga that you enjoy. Instead, you can use the practices in this book to complement the work you already do with your psychiatrist or psychologist. You can also integrate these practices directly into your psychotherapy sessions. You can continue to practice your preferred style of active yoga, and add these practices to it. Just make sure to integrate yoga's therapeutic elements into your life as much as you can.

While I was bringing yoga into psychotherapy and discovering session after session how much it helped people emotionally, a new field of yoga therapy began to emerge in full force in the West. Such venerated teachers as B. K. S. Iyengar and T. K. V. Desikachar and their senior students were implementing yoga therapy with people who suffered from a wide array of physical and psychological ailments. An International Association of Yoga Therapists (IAYT) was formed in 1989 and now has nearly three thousand members.

Many yoga therapists in this country today either focus exclusively on yoga therapy for physical issues, or use the philosophy of yoga to address mental and emotional issues such as anxiety or depression. My background as a clinical psychologist helps me to integrate the body-based *and* philosophical methods of yoga with decades of experience treating emotional imbalances. This fusion of yoga and psychotherapy has a profound impact on mental, physical, and emotional well-being.

It's no secret: healing emotional pain is a difficult endeavor. The World Health Organization expects that by the year 2030, depression will be the biggest health problem on our planet. The practices in this book are designed to counter the epidemics of anxiety and depression. I have fine-tuned them through many years of careful clinical observation and calibration. We have used them in classes, in workshops on the road, and in our center. They are universally accessible, easy to learn, and transformative. And yet, their effectiveness doesn't depend on a clinical setting or on the presence of an expert therapist. Rather, Integrative Yoga Therapeutics awakens your own ability to heal yourself. With practice, *you* can become your own yoga therapist.

My career began with a childhood desire to heal people. It grew into an adult mission to help people learn the skills they need to *heal themselves* throughout their lives. The practices in this book, together with your own hard work and persistence, can help you achieve emotional balance as well as the gift that lies just beyond it: deep fulfillment and happiness. I've seen it happen to many others, and it can happen to you as well.

Please consult a physician before beginning a Restorative Yoga practice if you are pregnant or have any of the following: a serious illness, eye pressure issues, back pain or a back injury, a detached retina, heart problems, serious skeletal injuries, lymphedema, or other illness. Although the postures in these sequences are gentle and safe by nature, it's still best to have medical approval before doing them. Bring this book to your doctor's office, as few physicians are likely to be familiar with Restorative Yoga.

Yoga for Emotional Balance

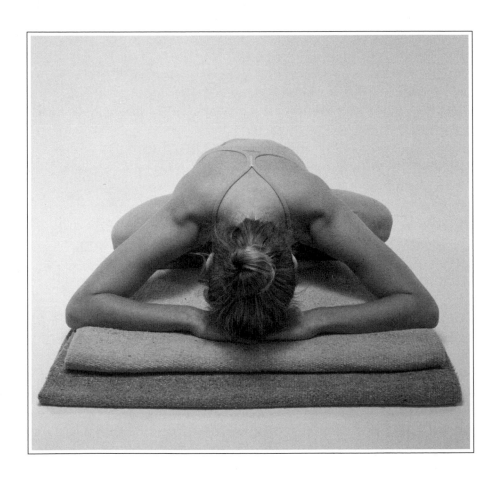

Introduction

Yoga's Role in Emotional Balance

You have the ability to live in emotional balance. What's more, it is your birthright. Yet life can get in the way. Chronic stress, multitasking, the pressure to have it all, and a value system that emphasizes achievement over self-care make emotional *imbalance*, not balance, more common in modern human experience.

Emotional imbalance can show up in many ways, such as low self-esteem, constant worrying, insomnia, persistent body-image issues, chronic pain disorders, or a general sense of malaise. It can stem from things like difficult family issues, abusive relationships, stressed-out parents, financial or social strain, and spiritual alienation. Yet no matter how it manifests, or what it stems from, emotional imbalance can be understood and changed. Imagine a continuum of emotional imbalance: at one end is anxiety, with racing thoughts, incessant worry, and physical agitation. At the other end is depression, with sluggish and negative thinking, lack of engagement in life, and physical lethargy. Where on that continuum does your mind lie? Where would your body be? As surprising as it sounds, the mind and body don't always echo one another. The interplay between them is so complex that the mind can occupy one end of the continuum while the body inhabits the other. Put another way, it's possible to experience both anxiety and depression at the same time.

This book is a guide to achieving emotional balance. If you struggle with occasional worry or gloom, it gives you tools to return to your emotional center. If you encounter periods of high stress or intense sadness, it provides practices to calm or rejuvenate you. If you suffer from regular, debilitating bouts of anxiety or depression that interfere with daily life, it offers you ways to rebuild your emotional health. And if you are a yoga therapist, yoga teacher, psychotherapist, or health-care professional, this book imparts a set of therapeutic tools that you can integrate into your practice.

The ideas in this book are rooted in the classical yoga tradition. They are supported by psychology and neuroscience. They are backed up by mind-body medicine and the emerging field of yoga therapy. They are brought to life by my clients and students who share their stories of struggle and healing. They offer new understanding about what strengthens your patterns of anxiety and depression, as well as practical tools you can use to change them.

These therapeutic tools include meditative practices, visualization, breathing exercises, relaxation techniques, and Restorative Yoga. They aren't complex: professional athletes, weekend warriors, yoga teachers, teachers-in-training, yoga students, and people brand-new to yoga have all used them successfully. Even if you've never set foot on a yoga mat, you too can practice them. As you do, you'll learn to navigate a wide range of emotional experiences without getting thrown off course. And ultimately, by connecting with your mind and body, you'll gain a glimpse of what lies beyond the emotional pain of anxiety and depression. Yoga opens a window to a new world. This world includes a connection to a deeper part of you that lives within and also transcends your mind and body: your spirit, or vital essence. But first, let's look at what emotional balance really means and how yoga can help you achieve it.

What Is Emotional Balance?

We are biologically primed for reaction; emotions are built into us. Few of us can encounter a dramatic display of anger without an answering burst of our own, or weather a romantic rejection without taking a hit to our self-esteem. Emotions aren't inherently bad;

even the most disruptive ones, like grief and anger, add richness and spice to our lives.

True emotional balance, then, is not about having only happy emotions. It has to do with how we *relate* to our emotions and to the residue they leave behind. After we've gone for the jugular with a sibling, for instance, can we reduce the angry aftereffects, or do we keep the fight alive? When our heart has been broken, how long does it take to restore our sense of self? When we're emotionally balanced, we experience and react to strong emotions such as fear, anger, sadness, or shame. We may even briefly immerse ourselves in them. Yet we're resilient: we refrain from drowning in our emotions or letting them limit us. And in the aftermath of a strong emotional reaction, we regulate our response and recover balance.

How Yoga Helps Create Emotional Balance

Not long ago, my brother-in-law intervened in one of my five-year-old nephew's emotional outbursts. My nephew was working up a full head of steam, entering that out-of-control zone from which children can take hours to return. What was my brother-in-law's clever remedy? He had his son stop, breathe deeply, and relax his body. Only minutes later, my nephew was in the sunroom playing quietly. Strange as it may sound, regulated breathing and relaxation are two keys to emotional balance; they help us handle strong emotions and recover from them. If my nephew, at his young age, can calm himself by breathing more deeply and relaxing his body, it's possible for anyone to do so.

In the West, the word *yoga* conjures up colorful images: hippies stretching amid clouds of incense, rows of athletic people sweating through yoga push-ups in a room heated to 103 degrees, yogis with their legs wrapped behind their heads, and trim suburban moms in tight-fitting yoga pants. These images can be off-putting. People often tell me, "Yoga isn't for me; I'm just not flexible." If you've counted yoga out, thinking that you're not strong enough, bendy enough, in shape enough, or *anything* enough, think again. To create emotional balance through yoga, you don't need flexibility or strength. You don't need to be young, full of energy, or in good physical health. You don't even need to be familiar with yoga. The simple practices chosen for this book center around two techniques: breathing and Restorative Yoga. These tools will help you become more body- and mind-aware, more relaxed, and more grounded in the present moment—which are all key elements of emotional balance. Let's look more closely at these tools and see how they work.

Breathing

Breathing seems so natural and ordinary; what could it possibly have to do with emotional balance? Breathing happens whether you think about it or not, so it doesn't receive the focus it deserves. Yet breath is our life force; without it, we can't exist. While we'd all agree that breath is necessary for survival and vitality, few people understand its impact on emotional health. Have you ever been engrossed in a suspenseful movie in which tension built over time and suddenly felt yourself exhale, only to realize you were holding your breath? Does that ever happen while you're driving in your car, working at your desk, or deep in a good book? Many people habitually hold their breath or breathe shallowly, even my advanced yoga students. It's possible to go through an entire yoga practice, or most of your life, without taking in or letting out a full breath.

But breathing has direct emotional consequences. Shallow, irregular breathing can increase heart rate, raise blood pressure, speed up the mind, and knock your nervous system out of balance. In contrast, regulated breathing can lower heart rate, decrease blood pressure, calm the mind, and bring your nervous system into balance. In other words, not breathing fully and deeply can make you more anxious or depressed, while regulated breathing can help to balance you. Yoga recognizes the power of breath, and gives it the prominence of its own special category of practice called *pranayama*, or breathwork. While some breathing exercises are best done on their own, the ones you'll find here can be integrated into practices such as Restorative Yoga, and even used in everyday life.

Restorative Yoga

Restorative Yoga originated in India in the twentieth century with B. K. S. Iyengar, founder of Iyengar Yoga, and his daughter Geeta. In

Restorative Yoga, the practitioner reclines in forward-bending (face-down) or back-bending (face-up) positions while fully supported by bolsters, blankets, and other props. B. K. S. Iyengar initially developed and prescribed these supported postures to help people with injuries, acute illness, and chronic disease.

Restorative Yoga doesn't burn hundreds of calories. It won't tone your abs. It won't give you the "yoga butt" that Hollywood has helped to advertise. And it doesn't resemble the high-intensity "yoga workout" that you might think is the only way to relieve your stress. Restorative Yoga is an internal practice. It benefits the mind and emotions just as much as the outer body, if not more. Restorative Yoga combines meditation and relaxation in a unique way: it quiets the mind and makes it more reflective, as meditation does. But the mind quiets *while* the body relaxes deeply, so reflection and insight become embodied.

Ideally, in the physical practice of yoga, our bodies develop a balance of strength and flexibility. Yet our minds crave similar equilibrium. Restorative Yoga emphasizes *mental* and *emotional* strength and flexibility, and gives our minds this balance. Through a restorative practice, we become strong enough to experience and tolerate a full range of feelings and then, with flexibility, return to a place of calm. The paradox? Although it does so much for us, Restorative Yoga can appear from the outside as though nothing much were happening. Because students are still, and supported by props, it can look passive, and even unexciting.

This is not to say that Restorative Yoga is easy—far from it. On the inside, it's alive, intense, challenging—a powerful *internal* practice. The hardest part, as I witness every Thursday night when I teach Restorative Yoga, is to be still. This is because when the body grows quiet, we can be faced with feelings we may have avoided. In other words, mental storms may come before the calm. Recently, ten minutes into a class, a woman flagged me down to ask if she could leave. "My mind's going so fast, I can't stand it," she explained. And at a weekend workshop not long ago, when a participant settled into his first restorative pose, the stress of his traumatic divorce threatened to overwhelm him. When the body slows down, the mind can accelerate as though it's practicing a fast-paced, strength-based, upside-down Ashtanga Yoga class. Week after week, I've watched people wrestle valiantly with the urge to get up, run around, and discharge the unsettling feelings that stillness can trigger. Yet if they can tolerate this initial discomfort, they create space for calm and for the emergence of a friendship between the mind and body.

Why Yoga Works

When we feel anxious or depressed, it's tempting to view our emotional difficulties as proof that we're unstable. I frequently hear people say, "I don't have what it takes to be happy," "I've been depressed all my life," or "I've always been anxious, as long as I can remember—I'll never learn to relax." This reaction to emotional pain is understandable, especially if it's been a long time since we've experienced anything different. But as we'll see in part 1, our emotional wiring—the way our brain cells are wired to communicate and respond to experience—may be locked onto the anxiety and depression settings. Therapeutic yoga can actually get deep enough into us to reset our emotional wiring. It gives us a new collection of tools that reverberate deep into the mind-body network. Yet how, exactly, does it do this?

The practice of yoga draws our focus from the world outside us (the one we're reacting to) and transfers it into the mind, brain, and body, where the roots of anxiety and depression lie. Naturally, we may want to escape our deep-seated issues as well as the pain of anxiety and depression. Yet through regulating the breath and relaxing the body, we learn to be *present* with our issues and our pain. We learn to resist getting caught up in our reactions, or letting them define us.

Beyond these benefits, therapeutic yoga offers something more. It gives us a firsthand, embodied experience of our fluctuating emotional landscapes. We can feel how emotions ebb and flow—how they really are short-lived, passing states of awareness. With even a brief interlude of not being anxious or depressed, we can begin to suspect that anxiety and depression *are not who we are;* they are just powerful emotional patterns that draw us in. We can replace these anxious or depressed emotional patterns with healthier ones.

Each year, our teacher-training program holds free group clinics for people with anxiety, depression, chronic pain, and other mind-body issues. For a seventy-five-minute span of time, our "guinea pigs," as we fondly think of them, are not anxious, depressed, or in pain. The changes are evident: Faces previously tense with anxiety are, during and after the practice, smoothed with calm. The slow, deadened movements and hunched posture of those with depression become infused with energy. The light that shines in their eyes afterward never fails to move me, though I see it every year.

Because yoga's experiential practices involve both the mind *and* the body, these insights and changes aren't simply mental; they are *embodied insights*, which tend to have a more lasting effect on anxiety and depression.

How to Use this Book

To gain the greatest benefit from this book, I suggest reading it from cover to cover. But I'd like to state upfront that the mental insights you'll find here, and beyond this book, are *not* the main instruments of change. You don't have to know how your mind and body work in anxiety and depression, though chapter 1 of this book discusses that. You don't need to know the three obstacles to emotional balance and why mental understanding alone doesn't work, though chapter 2 addresses those. It's not necessary to understand the mechanisms of true healing, though chapter 3 explores these issues. You can even get away without learning about the five key ways to transform your emotional patterns, which form the focus of chapter 4. And you can opt not to explore the greater meaning and opportunity that anxiety and depression offer, which is the theme of chapter 5. Yet without this knowledge, how can you change your emotional patterns and heal anxiety and depression?

Although knowledge is helpful, *practice* is the most important element in cultivating emotional balance. The exercises in this book (regulated breathing, restorative postures, developing mental focus, and learning to stay present with direct experience) re-wire your mind and body for improved emotional regulation. This means that you'll do better if you commit to doing the exercises at the end of each chapter in part 1, and those in part 2 regularly, and for an extended period of time. It's a good idea, at least in the beginning, to practice daily or several times weekly for a minimum of twelve weeks. Then practice regularly thereafter, to set your new wiring in place.

If you choose to skip the explanatory portions of this book and begin your therapeutic experience right away, I suggest that you start first with the exercises at the end of each chapter in part 1. These exercises aren't meant to be done once or twice to "get them right" and then move on. They're meant to be repeated over and over again to cultivate intelligence in the mind and body. They provide you with a solid foundation for the restorative sequences that come later. But they also work well on their own, so engage with them as often as you can. Once you feel confident about doing them, you can take the next step. You can identify your emotional type in chapter 6 (the first chapter in part 2), and then choose the sequence that best fits your type. While practicing the yoga routines in part 2, you might find it helpful to visit the earlier chapters at some point to gain a deeper understanding of anxiety and depression, how change best happens, and how breathing techniques and Restorative Yoga work.

This book also gives you access to audio recordings of some of the exercises in part 1 and the yoga routines in part 2. You can download these routines at www.shambhala.com/yogaforemotionalbalance, and listen to them whenever you prefer a guided practice.

It can feel like anxiety and depression are permanently wired into you, but they are not. Yet if you've suffered from anxiety and depression, why should you believe this? Neuroscientists are discovering how, with repeated practice of a skill or technique, the brain forges new neural networks. The mind, brain, and body, *and therefore our emotional patterns,* are capable of change. Without realizing it, you may have learned to reinforce your faulty wiring, to insulate yourself *against* emotional balance. Like all of us, you are an emotional electrician; you can learn to rewire yourself in healthier ways.

While it may feel as though you are alone, the yoga practices in this book help you develop a connection with your inner self that offers lifelong sustenance. When you discover this connection, you are no longer alone. Think of anxiety and depression as emotional rites of passage, opportunities in disguise. Each time they exert their pull, they provide you with a new opening to transcend your suffering and achieve emotional balance. They empower you to re-discover a potent natural resource: the healing interplay of mind, body, and spirit that already exists within you. They welcome you into the exciting and lifelong process of shifting and shaping the emotional patterns you may have thought were your destiny.

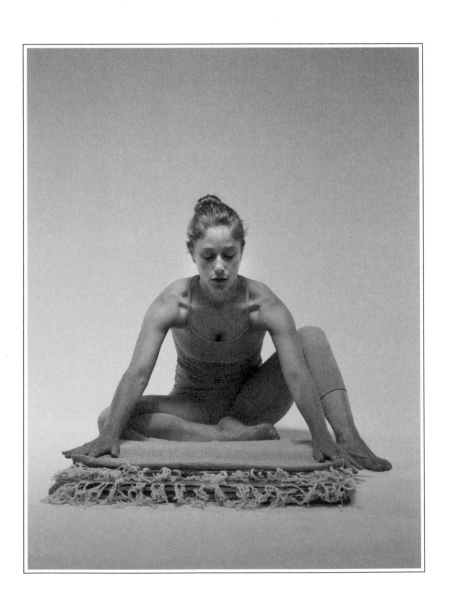

PART ONE

The Path to Emotional Balance

～1

Understanding Anxiety and Depression

A FEW YEARS AGO, AT THE START OF A WEEKEND WORKSHOP on yoga for anxiety and depression at Kripalu in Lenox, Massachusetts, I posed what I thought was an innocent, lighthearted question. Looking out over a sea of expectant faces I asked, "How many of you came here this weekend hoping to be healed?" Expecting chuckles or knowing nods, I was surprised to see nearly 100 percent of the participants raise their hands without a second thought. Their response made me think deeply about how we expect healing to happen.

People who read my articles or come to my classes, workshops, and retreats often tell me earnestly that yoga is their last hope. They know yoga can help them feel better, but can't quite grasp how. Meanwhile, they are bombarded by messages offering immediate gratification: "Eight weeks to a better body." "Lose ten pounds in five days!" The hard sell we get on emotional makeovers is no exception: "Feel better fast!" "Beat the blues!" This media deluge feeds an inner fantasy we all have of instant healing—a fantasy that doesn't take into account how many years we may have spent cultivating anxiety and depression.

In tough times we may wish for magic, for someone to take away our pain. Yet this magic does not exist. Even if it did, magical healing would deprive us of the growth that comes when we face our challenging emotional patterns and emerge victorious. The true medicine lies in going inward, in transforming the relationship we have with ourselves. Let's look more closely at this relationship, and see how it relates to emotional health.

The Mind-Body Network

Although the mind gets a lot of press for its role in emotional imbalance, anxiety (chronic or intense worry) and depression (long-term or acute sadness) are body issues as well. The mind *and* body feel the effects of anxiety and depression, and also contribute to them. This wouldn't matter as much if the mind and body weren't so closely connected. But thanks to an explosion of research in such fields as psychology, immunology, and neuroscience, we now know that the mind and body are inseparable. They are embedded within an elaborate infrastructure that shapes our response to emotions. This interplay of mind and body can make anxiety and depression feel insurmountable, but it can also be used to engender emotional balance.

The mind is the part of us that thinks, feels, and perceives. This includes the persona, the parts of ourselves that we show to others, and the private, inner parts. The mind constructs our conscious sense of being who we are: what yogis call the ego, or sense of "I am." The mind filters all our emotional experiences, such as happiness, worry, or sadness. Sometimes it does so in negative ways. It can paint us as "losers," the world as a difficult place, or life as having no meaning. Then it can grab onto these filtered emotional experiences and treat them as though they were true.

The mind's version of reality affects the body. The body, in turn, influences the mind. The body houses many systems that have a two-way relationship with our emotions: the heart and circulatory system, immune system, musculoskeletal system, endocrine system (which includes the glands that send and receive hormonal messages), and others. The body is also home to the nervous system, which plays a key role in anxiety, depression, and emotional well-being.

Just like the mind, the body affects the entire mind-body net-

work. Muscular tension, relaxation, changes in heart rate, and illness can interact with the mind and other emotional systems, and
contribute to anxiety and depression. This means that both the
mind and body participate in constructing positive or painful emotional experiences. Like musicians performing a duet, the mind and
body can compose countless variations on the themes of anxiety
and depression.

Both psychology and psychiatry have credited the mind with
more awareness and insight than the body. Yet my clients have
shown me that the body has its own powerful wisdom. Several
years ago Dierdre, a young dancer, came to me for a private session,
which was a birthday gift from her husband. At the beginning of
the session, I asked Dierdre to share her physical and emotional
goals. She quickly reassured me that emotionally, she was fine.
She'd lost touch with her core body, she said, and that's all she
wanted to work on. Yet her face, etched with tense lines of depression, said otherwise. Her body, shoulders sagging in defeat, agreed.
And as soon as Dierdre began to breathe in a simple seated posture, I noticed that her breath was shallow and irregular, as though
she couldn't allow herself to take in the gift of oxygen. We slowed
down and focused more closely on her breathing. I asked Dierdre to
lengthen her inhale, a seemingly minor adjustment. Almost immediately, her eyes welled up with tears. It turned out that her body
had held on to grief from her mother's death one year earlier, and
was waiting faithfully until she had time to address it. Most likely,
this was the first deep connection with her direct experience that
she'd allowed herself in months.

The body feels emotions, too. It speaks its pain as clearly as the
mind—just not verbally. Even in psychotherapy, when a client sits
fairly still, it's possible to read the interplay of emotions throughout
the body. Anxiety can seem to lie coiled like a spring underneath
the skin, while the heavy weight of depression can sink someone's
shoulders and chest. Our body often broadcasts the very vulner-
abilities that we try so hard to hide.

Both the mind *and* the body respond to emotional experience.
Both are sentient. Their intelligence plays a key role in keeping anxiety and depression alive, and an equally significant role

in healing. A closer look at anxiety and depression will show us how this mind-body intelligence works in action. See if you recognize yourself in the descriptions below. That way, when we get to part 2 of this book, you'll have a head start on identifying your emotional type.

How Your Mind and Body Wire Anxiety

What do racing thoughts, an elevated heart rate, and fast physical movements have in common? All three are ways that your mind and body indicate and also "build" on anxiety. Your mind provides the sped-up, worried thoughts. Your nervous system builds on that foundation by elevating heart rate and blood pressure and producing a host of other mind-body effects. Your body chimes in with rapid physical movements, or fidgeting, that add to the overall experience of anxiety. When the mind, nervous system, and body act in unison, their small contributions have big effects on your emotional well-being.

Here's how this works in greater detail. When your mind builds anxiety, your thoughts accelerate. They become lightning-fast, incessant, and full of worry. Anxious thoughts focus primarily on the future: *What if my boss isn't happy with this project? Will my wife be home on time tonight? What if he's still angry with me?* Because you can't control future events, your worry gains an out-of-control intensity. Even something as small as a change in someone's facial expression can trigger a fresh round of worry. You become more sensitive to the tiniest nuances of your environment, which leaves you vulnerable to further anxious reactions, and so on. The part of your mind-body network that tells you there's nothing to worry about is often slow to respond. This explains why, in the midst of a fight with a loved one, you might feel your heart race, your palms sweat, and your stomach drop to the floor. It accounts for why those feelings can persist for hours, or even days, after the fight is over. The part of the mind that interprets experience seizes upon any whisper of uncertainty in your environment and amplifies it. What's more, telling others about your worrisome events or interactions can intensify not just your anxiety, but theirs.

Your body helps wire in anxiety, too. When you are feeling anxious, your movements can become more rapid, as though driven from within, and you may find it hard to slow down. You may struggle to be fully present in your body, which makes it difficult to realize how fast or erratically you're moving. In my national workshops, I ask my assistant teachers to demonstrate what anxiety and depression look like in a yoga practice. We've affectionately nicknamed these movements "Whippets" after the lightning-fast dogs at the racetrack, and this is by far the most popular of our demonstrations. The anxiety "models" begin by scanning the room frenetically and fidgeting in place. As I start to instruct a sequence of Sun Salutations (part of the beginning sequence of the Vinyasa Yoga practice), they move so fast that they nearly give themselves whiplash. They can't slow down, so they stay five steps or poses ahead of my directions. Transitions from one pose to the next are rapid, and done without any sense of alignment. This demonstration always earns a chorus of laughs, beet-red faces, and knowing nods from workshop participants, who recognize these signs of agitation in themselves.

After the demonstration, we often ask workshop participants to experiment by exaggerating anxiety in their own minds and bodies. We take them through a round or two of superfast Whippet Sun Salutations, with such rapid movements and so few transitions that their breathing becomes shallow and rapid. This intensifies anxiety, as we'll discuss in the chapters that follow. They also scan the room rapidly with their eyes and try to stay attuned to everything going on around them. At the end of three minutes, they feel "amped-up," "anxious," and "hyper." We always have them follow this exercise with 1:2 Breathing (page 72) to calm and balance their self-induced anxiety. This exercise gives the participants an embodied awareness of how posture, movement, and nervous system activation can create or worsen anxiety. It then makes more sense to them when we introduce regulated breathing, mindful movement, and restorative postures (the opposite of Whippets) as therapeutic tools to balance anxiety.

If you fall on the anxiety end of the emotional balance continuum, you may be in a state of constant physical agitation, as

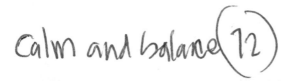

Calm and balance (72)

though a motor were racing inside you. Throughout the first year of his yoga practice, Frank continually moved his toes as though conducting an inaudible symphony. This was his body's way of expressing anxiety during the final Relaxation Pose (the one in which practitioners close their eyes, adjust their breath, and relax their bodies). The stillness of the pose highlighted his anxiety, and his movements helped discharge it. Like Frank, people with physical symptoms of anxiety often benefit from grounding and "enclosed" poses to conserve energy and redirect their focus inward. These are Restorative Yoga's forward-bending or "neutral" poses (see chapter 8). They also respond well to regulated breathing, especially 1:2 Breathing, to calm the mind (see chapter 3).

How Your Mind and Body Wire Depression

How do your mind and body collaborate to create and build on depression? They might take disappointment or rejection as a starting point. Your mind can filter the disappointment negatively, deciding that it has something to do with you. Your thoughts move slowly, and you're likely to ruminate on what's happened in a negative, self-blaming way: *Why did he have to leave me? No one will ever love me like that again. Why am I such a loser?* This uses up so much of your mind's juice that it can feel as though your mental power cable has been shut off. You may be convinced that you'll never feel better, that you're helpless to change your life. At this point, your mind may interpret new experiences, even positive ones, in a more pessimistic light.

The myopic nature of the depressed mind is largely blind to positive experiences, and allows mostly negative ones into your line of vision. Just as an anxious mind can filter experiences as threatening or worrisome, a depressed mind sees them as deflating or depressing. Nelle, a young associate of mine, is currently a member of what I'd call the "Worst Lives Club." When you ask Nelle how she's doing, she'll say that she's one day away from a demotion (she has a highly successful position in a prestigious consulting firm). She believes her female mentor exploits her (she actually has a nurturing boss). She magnifies her boyfriend's occasional forgetfulness or spacing out into enormous transgressions (he's really quite attentive). Not surprisingly, Nelle surrounds herself with friends who share her doom-and-gloom perspective. Their conversations sound like contests to determine who has the worst work or personal life. She doesn't realize, however, that the grand prize is something she doesn't want: depression. Nelle's negative way of viewing the world, and the social mileage she gets from it, only feed her depression. She hasn't taken up yoga yet because, as she says, "Nothing I've tried has helped, so I doubt yoga will, either."

Your body also contributes to the foundation of depression. When you're depressed, your body feels lethargic and tired. You may become so preoccupied that your body gets "lost" in space, and even simple movements can become challenging. When my assistant teachers demonstrate how depression is reflected in the physical practice of yoga, they allow their bodies to release any core muscle engagement and sink toward the ground with heaviness. Their yawning and fatigue become contagious, and I often hear the audience sighing and beginning to yawn themselves. The "depressed practitioners" are withdrawn; they delay each movement, and make the transitions between poses tentative and lethargic. This leaves them only two-thirds of the way through their Sun Salutations when my instructions have finished. After the demonstration, workshop participants often comment how tired and devoid of energy they feel just from watching.

Depression can imprint not only your movement patterns, but your posture as well. Your body may have what I call "Closed Heart Syndrome," a postural pattern that illustrates the helplessness, hopelessness, and self-protective withdrawal of depression. In Closed Heart Syndrome, the chest sinks and the heart area collapses. This makes the breath shallow and slow; we'll discuss the effects of shallow breathing in the chapters that follow. The upper spine and shoulders round, as though to protect the heart from further disappointment. This also protects us from intimacy, which people with depression may see as merely another chance to be hurt. In workshops, we sometimes have participants emulate

Closed Heart Syndrome for one minute. After only twenty seconds, some ask to stop. Sixty seconds in, and they report feelings of sadness, fatigue, and hopelessness. This helps them internalize how postural patterns can contribute to or worsen depression. It gives them a context for why we use head and neck alignment, heart-opening restorative postures, and deep breathing to lift and balance depression. People who have physical symptoms of depression often benefit from opening the upper thoracic spine and chest areas. The best postures for them are the back-bending Restorative Yoga postures (see chapter 9). An equal breath ratio or 1:1 Breathing (page 48) helps keep the mind balanced yet alert.

Posture and movement can be insidious in building anxiety and depression. Without realizing it, we repeat physical patterns hundreds of times daily, sharpening them on the whetstone of our experience. Certain patterns, such as whippet movements or closed-heart syndrome, can exacerbate anxiety or depression. These patterns add to the emotional pain that we've tried so hard to lessen.

Crossed Wiring: What Happens in Mixed Anxiety and Depression

Recently, as I was channel surfing between innings of a Red Sox game, a commercial took me by surprise. Before I knew consciously what the product was, I heard the dramatic musical overture favored by pharmaceutical companies. A distraught, lank-haired, haunted-eyed woman slumped tiredly against a wall in the background. The commercial's opening words established its unique pitch: to boldly go where no other commercial had gone before and challenge the effectiveness of antidepressants.

"Two-thirds of all people on antidepressants," intoned the announcer, "do not get better." I watched, stunned, at full attention. Accompanied by the merry strains of musical resolution and a view of the now-happy, fluffy-haired protagonist, the announcer went on to trumpet the benefits of a new antidepressant called Abilify *when used in combination with other antidepressants.* To me, the real news was not the launching of Abilify. It was the public acknowledgment that antidepressants often fail to significantly improve symptoms of depression for *most people.* Why might this happen, and what can we do about it?

There may be many reasons why antidepressants are less effective than we'd like. One, however, has to do with how the mind and body wire *mixtures* of anxiety and depression, rather than just one or the other, into us. Ayurveda, yoga's system of medicine, recognizes that *the symptoms your mind experiences can differ from the ones your body feels.* The mind, for example, can be highly anxious (with rapid and worried thoughts) while at the same time, the body can be slowed-down and lethargic. On the other hand, the body can be physically agitated and much too energized, while the mind functions slowly and with difficulty.

This division makes excellent clinical sense. Throughout my years as a psychologist, I've worked with many people who took medication to manage symptoms of anxiety or depression. Medication usually "took the edge off" and helped them function better. In some cases, however, the results were not what we expected. Anti-anxiety medications sometimes calmed the mind, but at the same time made the body too lethargic. On the other hand, antidepressant medications often increased physical energy, but triggered racing thoughts and mental anxiety. In response, doctors frequently prescribed an additional medication to manage the side effects of the first one. This proved challenging for my clients; many took medication only with reluctance, and strongly disliked taking more than one. In my opinion, this multimedication approach is a little like training a dog by telling it, "Go, fetch!" and "Stay, sit!" at the same time. People who suffer from a mixture of anxiety and depression often receive this "contradictory training" with medication. What's worse, studies show that people with *mixed* anxiety and depression tend to take more medications, and improve to a lesser extent, than people with *either* anxiety *or* depression.

In my early years as a yoga therapist, I saw something similar with my yoga clients. Many wanted to address their anxiety and depression without taking medication. For most of them, the breathing exercises and restorative sequences for anxiety and depression worked well. Yet in some, I saw what I'd seen as a psychologist:

a certain percentage with anxiety, when practicing calming yoga techniques, became too low in energy. Others with depression, when practicing mood-lifting breathwork and restorative poses, experienced a surge of dormant mental anxiety.

This happened with Gary, a yoga student who suffered from depression. Gary's body had significant lethargy and tiredness, and he complained of a steady thirty-pound weight gain. His mind, on the other hand, worried incessantly and focused obsessively on every change in his surroundings. Work was particularly difficult for him: the prospect of an upcoming meeting could send his thoughts into overdrive. He couldn't press pause on his persistent mental videos, which featured his boss firing him in front of all his colleagues.

How would modern medicine treat Gary? Most likely with psychotherapy and perhaps also an antidepressant. In fact, that's just what happened. Before coming to see me, Gary had tried three different antidepressants but found it difficult to tolerate the increased mental activity—which he described as "agitation"—that accompanied them. When his doctor prescribed an anti-anxiety medication to calm his mind, Gary had an adverse reaction to the drug. He felt frustrated; he wanted to manage his depression holistically, without using medication.

Because of the history and symptoms he presented, I felt that Gary had depression in his body and anxiety in his mind, or "Anxious Depression" (for more information on "Anxious Depression" and its converse, "Depressed Anxiety," see "Emotional Type 3: Depressed Body/Anxious Mind" and "Emotional Type 4: Anxious Body/Depressed Mind, in chapter 6). In people with Anxious Depression, like Gary, treatment that targets the body's depressive symptoms and increases physical energy can cause agitation and racing thoughts in the mind. I had Gary try the "Balancing Mixed Anxiety and Depression" practice (presented in chapter 10), which combines physically energizing restorative poses with mentally calming breathwork. After several weeks of practice, Gary reported less lethargy and depression in his body. And due to the breathing exercises, his mind felt balanced and calm, punctuated only by the infrequent bursts of anxiety that most of us encounter. His mental videos no longer felt so compelling. He worried less about getting fired, and could work with greater focus and concentration.

Yoga can address the mind and body at the same time. When necessary, it can even treat the mind and body in different ways. This makes it an ideal practice for people with anxiety, depression, *and* mixed anxiety-depression, as well as for people who fluctuate between anxiety and depression. For example, on days when you find that your mind is anxious and your physical energy is low, like Gary's, you can create a practice that calms your mind and thoughts but energizes your body.

The Myth of Instant Healing

Whether we've suffered from anxiety or depression for as long as we can remember, or occasionally hit pockets of emotional turbulence, many of us yearn for "instant healing." We may secretly hope that the right therapist or experience will immediately unlock a magical cure, banishing our emotional challenges to the past and turning us into the fearless and healthy people we've always wanted to be. Suddenly, we'll be the assertive woman with healthy boundaries who doesn't give her power away to others. We'll be the woman who on the heels of a romantic rejection gets up, dusts herself off, says "It's his loss," and continues to believe in romantic love. We'll turn into the confident guy whose self-esteem remains steady through fortunate *and* disappointing events. We'll be the guy who succeeds at a job that actually interests him, and never obsesses over his bald spot. We'll be free of the self-defeating habits, the mental scorecard of ancient grievances, the "emotional snowball" that makes it so hard to forgive ourselves and others. We'll be an emotional Wonder Woman or Superman. We'll be invulnerable. This is the fantasy—the myth—of instant healing.

Mike, a graduate student in his late twenties, fell prey to this fantasy. Mike suffered from a deep depression. He took antidepressants and saw a wonderful therapist every week, but still felt that his quality of life was intolerable. He often missed work due to low energy and lack of motivation, and his last two relationships ended when his girlfriends decided he was "too high-maintenance." Mike came to one of my weekend workshops on yoga for depression. He'd never done yoga before, but during the weekend he embraced the concept that his body was a vehicle for healing. He participated in each practice session wholeheartedly. Toward the end of the Saturday morning heart-opening class, Mike felt a new sense of expansion in his body. With each successive yoga technique, he gained more energy and greater hope. He *felt* the connection between deeper breathing and present-moment awareness. He *sensed* how balancing his nervous system led to greater emotional well-being. He *experienced* the link between being present in his body and increased positive emotions. I warned the workshop participants that these new experiences (in particular, the postural adjustments that align the spine and bring more energy into the body, the breathing exercises that expand lung capacity and balance the mind, and the restorative sequences that lift depression) needed to be practiced repeatedly for lasting change to occur. As I looked out into the audience, Mike jokingly put his hands over his ears and grinned. All kidding aside, I could see that he felt he was healed. His experiences made him feel that his life had changed, permanently, for the better. He left the weekend on an "instant-healing high."

Expecting his ten-hour weekend experience to take care of everything, Mike returned home and didn't practice again. He was shocked when, after one week, he couldn't get out of bed. His body felt drained of energy, and the door in his heart felt like it was closing. He began to dwell again on all the things that seemed wrong with his life. Even the burning out of a lightbulb in his bedroom felt as if the world were trying to punish him. This time, Mike's despondency was aggravated by the conviction that he'd done something to ruin his newfound healing. He felt he just didn't "deserve for the good feelings to stick around."

A few weeks later, Mike contacted the Center for Integrative Yoga Therapeutics, our yoga therapy center in Boston, with a request for private sessions. With time, he realized that the disappearance of his "yoga miracle" was neither his fault, nor was it about deserving to feel better; it was simply a natural consequence of not practicing. Mike went to yoga therapy each week and practiced restorative postures on his own several times weekly. After six months, he regained most of the progress he'd made during the transformative weekend. More importantly, he grasped one of the essential "rules" of how change happens. Any healing practice, including yoga, is meant to build over a lifetime, and not simply be practiced once or twice, to realize its full effect. And that wasn't all. "Something weird happened," Mike said, in the half-year process of healing. He gained a sense of the ebb and flow of his emotions. He began to feel a friendship with himself. He developed a faith that he had what it takes to be emotionally resilient—all things that "instant healing" hadn't given him.

When we emphasize the *outcome* of our personal growth work over the *process*, we deny ourselves an important gift. Healing through slow, steady work enhances our self-esteem. It gives us the conviction that we can tackle anything. When we focus on healing progressively, we embrace the idea that we evolve throughout our lives. We begin to understand that the process of evolution is as healing as the outcome.

Each time we pick up a self-help book, sign up for a workshop, or make an appointment with a new doctor or healer, we're filled with anticipation. *This is it,* we may think: the experience we've been waiting for. Certainly, a workshop, retreat, or class can make us feel better. Yet when we think the magic has kicked in, we may excuse ourselves from the "grunt work," from the effort of daily practice. This also happened to Esmee, a yoga student of mine. With her doctor's supervision, Esmee used yoga therapeutics to help her taper off antidepressants. "I did it!" she told me excitedly. Yet when I asked her what her yoga "maintenance plan" was, she looked at me strangely. "Why do I need that?" she asked. "I'm better!"

Beauty magazines, Hollywood movies, and reality-TV shows all tout the dramatic effects of a makeover. Yet they rarely reveal what it takes to maintain quick improvements. When those improvements either sputter at the start or whither from lack of nourishment or continued practice, we can lose hope. We're likely to leave that new book half-read or put it back on the shelf. We may give up on workshops (or sign up for different ones). We may despair of ever feeling better. The instant healing fantasy can cause a backlash: we may find ourselves drawn back into old patterns, which can make us feel even worse. In over two decades of work with people who suffer from anxiety and depression, I've observed that the desire for instant change—and the tendency to give up when we don't find it—is one of the main reasons why people fail to get better.

I don't want this to happen to you. Together, we can avoid it. We can explore the brain's capacity for change. We can learn that instant healing flies in the face of what we know about how our brains are wired, and we can spend time investigating how true healing actually occurs. We can acknowledge that true healing requires regular, continued, and *specific* practices that build over time. And we can engage with these healing practices in a long-term, committed relationship.

How Yoga Creates Change

If you've tried for a long time to "fix" your anxiety and depression through medication or psychotherapy, these are not your only options. You can add yoga to any treatment you're currently using and see beneficial effects. Unlike medication and psychotherapy, yoga addresses the mind *and* body at the same time. Yoga's physical poses (both active and restorative) help build new body experiences that differ from anxiety and depression. This tells every system in your mind-body network that you are not anxious and not depressed. Yoga also influences posture: it can shift the very movement and alignment patterns that have led to a closed heart area, amped-up muscular tension, or sped us up to the point of agitation.

Yoga's benefits don't stop there. Its special breathing techniques can calm an anxious mind or invigorate a sluggish one. Its use of relaxation, after each practice and in restorative poses, balances the nervous system. And yoga's ability to help us attend to our direct experience (sometimes called present-moment awareness), as we will see, also sets the stage for quieting the mind and changing mental patterns. Yoga's therapeutic tools (focused attention, visualization, breathing exercises, relaxation, and Restorative Yoga, to name a few) don't just begin to assemble new, healthier emotional experiences. They reach beyond these experiences to the root of our original suffering: a separation from the deepest parts of ourselves, which we will explore further in chapter 5.

Yoga is mind-body medicine. It works through the mind and body to help heal anxiety, depression, and other forms of emotional pain. Promising new developments in yoga research support this claim. Here are just a few ways that yoga can improve our awareness, posture, and mood: After practicing yoga, people with eating disorders experienced greater body awareness, more positive feelings about their bodies, and healthier attitudes toward food and eating.[1] Sitting upright helped people generate positive thoughts, while slumping made negative thoughts more compelling.[2] After a physical yoga practice, participants reported decreased levels of anxiety, depression, and feelings of anger.[3] And yogic breathing can increase resilience to stress and reduce anxiety, depression, and post-traumatic stress disorder.[4]

Despite yoga's many promising benefits, change is still difficult. What do we need to do to ensure that nothing gets in the way of creating and reinforcing healthier emotional experiences? The chapter that follows will reveal three main influences that can slow down *or speed up* the healing process—and yoga happens to address all three.

About the Exercises in this Book

At the end of chapters 1–5 (part 1) of this book, you will find a breathing exercise and a body exercise. Each exercise includes three parts: First, you'll get your "baseline" by determining how you feel before beginning. Second, you'll do the exercise, being as present as possible. Third, you'll feel the difference, comparing how you felt before the exercise to how you feel after it, to help you measure its effects. Practicing in this way helps you become more attuned to the effects of subtle practices such as breathing and cultivating body awareness. Your observations are self-discoveries. Consider using a journal to record any observations you make during these exercises. Your journal also chronicles your growth and change, and you may choose to revisit it later for inspiration.

All of the breathing exercises in this book are designed to bring awareness to your breath. If you tend to breathe mostly through your mouth, you may need to spend several sessions just training yourself to breathe in and out through your nose. The same is true if you've been taught to inhale through your nose but exhale through your mouth. Nasal breath (for both the inhale and the exhale) is an important tool in creating emotional balance. Please make sure that you're comfortable with breathing in *and* out through your nose before you start any of the exercises in this book.

 ## Breath Exercise: Getting to Know Your Breath

This exercise, Getting to Know Your Breath, marks the beginning of using your breath as a tool to balance your emotions. Here, you'll simply observe your breath without trying to change it in any way.

Get Your Baseline

Find a quiet space where you can spend at least five minutes un-interrupted. This time is just for you; it's *your* time to become acquainted with your breath. Sit in any comfortable position for you: in a chair, on the floor with a cushion supporting you, or with your back resting against a wall. If you don't find sitting comfortable, you can also lie down on your back with your knees bent. It may sound strange, but many of us have never gotten to know our breath before; most of us haven't begun the practice of connecting our breath with our mood.

In order to measure the effectiveness of this breath technique in balancing your emotions, you need to establish your baseline—in other words, how your body and mind feel right now. Since breath affects your mind and brain most quickly, take your mental base-line first. It may help to close your eyes. What's going on in your mind now? Are your thoughts moving fast, flitting from one thing to the next? Are they slow and sleepy? Or are they somewhere in the middle? Are your thoughts focused on the future (more like anxiety) or on past events (more like depression)? It may help to use a 1–10 scale, with "1" being slow thoughts and "10" representing a racing mind. Or you can just note something like "fast mind" or "sluggish mind."

Now take a baseline of your body's energy level. Use the same 1–10 scale, with "1" representing extreme physical lethargy and "10" representing intense energy, almost to the point of feeling hyperactive. Write down your mental and physical baselines so you can compare them to how you feel afterward. Getting your baselines will help you be more aware of the effects of this breathing exercise.

Do the Practice

Continue to sit as before, or if you wish, change your sitting posture so that you can sit comfortably; if possible, place a rug or something soft underneath you. If sitting upright doesn't feel good right now, use a folded blanket beneath you to elevate your hips and sit with your back against the wall and your head resting gently against it. If you like, you can also lie on your back with your knees bent.

Slowly close your eyes. Allow the closing of your eyes to signal your mind and body that you are moving from an outer-directed to an inner-directed awareness. This inner-directed awareness is one of the keys to emotional balance, and you can practice it every time you do one of these exercises, or even on its own. It's possible to close your eyes, and still maintain tension or activity in your eyeballs, which is not ideal. Allow your eyeballs to relax. Visualize them moving inward, dropping gently toward your heart. In this way, your outer sight—the awareness that focuses on things outside of you—becomes inner sight, or *in*sight.

Begin to breathe in and out through your nose for about one minute. When you are ready, start counting the length of your breath. Let each count be about one second. You don't need to be completely accurate when counting seconds. Just get a good approximation that you can use consistently to measure the length of your breath. Let your breath be natural, and not forced. As you breathe, imagine that you are directing your breath upward, to the level of your eyes. Inhale and feel your ribs expanding on the front of your body. Exhale fully. Do this several times. Then inhale again, and feel your side and back ribs fill and expand, almost as though they're smiling. Allow your abdomen to relax. As you focus on your breath, release any judgmental thoughts or worries that you are not "doing it right." Instead, observe your breath calmly and without judgment.

Continue to breathe in and out through your nose. If it helps, count as you breathe in and count as you breathe out. Notice how many counts it takes to breathe in and how many counts it takes to breathe out. Remember this number if you can—or write it down in your notes before continuing. Once you've counted your inhale and exhale, continue to breathe without counting.

If you are able to, begin to lengthen both your inhale and your exhale; see whether you can increase them by just one count. If this feels uncomfortable, return to a count that is more natural to you. When approximately five minutes have passed, return to your normal breathing pattern for a minute or two. Then slowly open your eyes.

Be as compassionate as you can about the length of your breath. Even if you've had difficulty with this exercise, there's good news: regulating your breath is one of those skills that develops very quickly with practice. Your breath may seem shallow or short to you now, but take heart: it will improve dramatically with time and practice.

Feel the Difference

Before you continue reading or turn to any other activities that might be clamoring for your attention, take several moments to *feel the difference.* Notice any change between the mental and physical baselines you had before, and how you feel right now. Has your mind slowed down? Do you feel calmer? Have your thoughts evened out or slowed down a little, or are they more balanced now between fast and slow?

Check in with your body: Does it feel somewhat more relaxed?

Note any improvements or changes in your journal. Don't worry if at first you can't pinpoint a difference. As time goes on, you'll become more and more adept at taking your mental and emotional "temperature" and observing your response to these exercises.

Note your own personal "breath style" in your journal or on a piece of paper. At your starting point, how many counts were your inhale and exhale? Which was longer? Over time, you can work on lengthening both—or the shorter one—to build up your breath capacity.

Body Exercise: Distinguishing between Tension and Relaxation

Get Your Baseline

In this exercise, you'll begin the process of becoming more at home in your body, one of the most important prerequisites for calming your nervous system and creating emotional balance. Take your physical baseline: How relaxed or tense do you feel? Do you have areas of chronic physical tension? If so, where are they? The neck, shoulders, back, and abdomen are typical places where physical tension or tightness occur. If you're not sure whether you have physical tension, note that, too.

As you connect more with your body, you'll be able to feel more clearly the difference between physical tension and relaxation. This way, when you begin to use the practices later in this book, you'll have a baseline to which you can compare your growing capacity for relaxation. You'll also learn about where your body stores tension. Then you can use your breath and awareness to release that tension whenever you wish.

Do the Practice

Sit in a comfortable chair or lie down. (Keep in mind, however, that if you lie down, you may have trouble staying awake!) Slowly close your eyes. Begin to breathe in and out through your nose. Turn your awareness inward, and draw it further in with each inhale.

As you breathe, tighten the skin on your forehead by raising your eyebrows and smiling widely at the same time. Tighten your mouth and jaw and neck. You can squint your eyes, scrunch your face into a tiny ball, or do anything you need in order to tighten your facial muscles. Notice what happens to your breathing. Can you still breathe easily? As your body tightens, you may find that your breathing simultaneously becomes shallow.

Continue to feel the tightness or stuck energy in your body. What does this tightness feel like? Is it unfamiliar to you? Or has it been with you so long that you hardly notice its presence? Sometimes it's possible to be so busy that you don't inhabit your body very often. If this is the case, you may have difficulty going inward, or be surprised at how much tension you carry.

Now completely relax your eyes, face, head, and neck. Breathe in and out through your nose as you experience the sensation of relaxation. Notice the difference between the tightness you felt just a few moments ago and the relaxation you feel now.

Bring your awareness to your hands. Ball your hands into fists and keep them tight. Again, notice your breathing. Is it hard to breathe while you clench your fists? Hold for a few breaths and then release the tension and contraction. Next, direct your breath into your hands. Feel the difference between now and the tension you felt just a few moments ago. Note that just as you were capable of producing tension, you're also capable of creating relaxation. In fact, you're doing it right now. Don't worry if you can't yet feel any difference; your awareness will develop with time and regular practice.

Next, focus on your abdomen. Contract your abdominal muscles and draw your navel sharply toward your spine. Once again, notice your breath. How much more difficult is it to breathe when your abdomen is tense? Many people have persistent abdominal tension; perhaps you hold tension there, too. Release your muscles completely and deepen your breath. Using your visualization skills, imagine that you are drawing your breath into your abdomen to help it relax.

Repeat this exercise with as many body parts as you wish: your arms, legs, feet, shoulders. Each time, notice what the tension feels like. Notice what happens to your breath in response to the tension. And then feel the difference in your breath and your body when you release that tension.

When you are ready to stop, breathe normally, in and out through your nose, for several minutes. Then slowly open your eyes.

Feel the Difference

Before continuing on to the next chapter or exercise, spend some time comparing the "before" and "after" sensations. Look back in your journal to see where you felt tension before beginning the exercise. Did the tension dissipate as you progressed through the exercise? Note whether you feel less tension, or even full relaxation, in those areas now.

How has this progressive relaxation and breathing exercise changed your body and your mind? Do you feel more relaxed? How does your mind feel? Are your thoughts slower or calmer? If you have difficulty pinpointing a difference, don't be concerned. As time goes on, it will get easier to feel and observe your response to these exercises. As hard as it may be to believe this right now, "small" practices such as these have a big impact on your mood and your ability to regulate your emotions, so do them as often as you can.

⌒2

What Gets in the Way
of Change

DO YOU EVER BEGIN A CONVERSATION WITH SOMEONE close to you with the best of intentions, knowing where the mine-fields lie and resolving to take the high road, only to find your-self becoming agitated and angry within minutes? Have you ever vowed to begin a new romantic relationship with good boundaries, and then given so much that you lose all sense of who you are? Changing emotional patterns is a difficult endeavor. It has little to do with motivation, or even insight. It has everything to do with what kind of experiences we have most of the time, and how they influence our wiring.

The conscious mind frequently recognizes that negative patterns hurt us. Often, we even know what we need to do about them. Yet despite this recognition, things can stubbornly stay the same. Many of the wisest, most perceptive people I know work hard to make the changes they desire, yet lasting change often eludes them. The complaints that have sounded most loudly in my ears include: "Everything's great when I'm talking to you here in the office, but a few hours later, I'm right back where I started"; "I know what I need to do, but I just can't seem to do it"; "I've got every reason to be happy, but that doesn't change how I feel"; and "I know I need to relax, but stress gets in my way."

A Grand Canyon–sized gap exists between knowing what to do

and doing it, between mental understanding and the real-life experience of change. As a psychologist and yoga therapist, I've spent a good deal of time contemplating this gap. Why does it exist? Why can't hard-won insight or a good yoga class immediately transform us? The answer is simple: the mind-body network constantly patterns and refines our emotional experiences in a particularly powerful way. Whether we're aware of it or not, this network uses repetition to strengthen the patterns of anxiety and depression.

Why Do We Get Stuck in a Rut?

Psychology and yoga philosophy each study the formation of habits through repetition. Both seem to agree that we are born with and also develop a menu of exceptionally powerful patterns: mental, emotional, neural (related to the wiring in our brain), physical, and behavioral. In yogic terms, these patterns are known as *samskaras*. The word *samskara* comes from the Sanskrit *sam* ("complete" or "joined together") and *kara* ("action," "cause," or "doing"). Our samskaras make up our habits, our conditioning. Psychology would call this "repetition compulsion." Yet both terms indicate that the toughest negative patterns can compel us so strongly that we have almost no choice but to repeat them. Each repetition engraves an anxiety or depression samskara more deeply into our consciousness.

Samskaras can be positive: we might make a habit of acknowledging mistakes, accepting accountability for our actions, or honoring our own and others' needs. They can also be negative: we may mount an offensive attack rather than admit we're wrong, blame others for our actions, or serve others' needs to the exclusion of our own.

We are creatures of habit: the mind, body, and other emotional systems all naturally incline toward patterns. This is because our bodies, brains, and nervous systems are designed to maintain homeostasis—to keep things the same—even when we wish they wouldn't. In an anxiety pattern, for instance, the nervous system incessantly sounds the alarm, although we know intellectually that there's nothing to worry about. In a depression samskara, our self-concept might stubbornly gravitate toward self-disgust or shame, despite constant reassurance from people who love us.

Many of my students are quick to see the negative potential in samskaras. They assume them to be bad and resolve to "get rid of" them. Yet there's no escaping samskaras. Most of us cycle through certain ones over and over throughout our lives. These become our "signature samskaras." Yet when we do the hard work of self-study and becoming present, we cultivate different, less destructive, and healthier patterns.

The Body Contributes to Emotional Pain

Like all elements of the mind-body network, the body participates in creating emotional patterns. I recently taught on yoga for anxiety at a national conference where Peter, one of the participants, demonstrated this well. In Downward Dog Pose, Peter drove his shoulders and head aggressively toward the mat. With each breath, he bounced his body farther toward the floor, ignoring the loud signals of neck and upper-back tension that had caused him nearly two years of suffering. He expressed great interest and comprehension when I showed him how this pattern of movement—of forcing an action that his body couldn't safely do—created chronic neck pain. He really seemed to get how this chronic pain and stiffness increased his anxiety. I showed Peter how to lift his head and shoulders away from the floor, engage his core muscles, release his neck, and allow his entire body to participate equally in the pose. He practiced this new way of doing the pose with relief, and even remarked how great it felt. Yet a few poses later, he was back to his old Downward Dog. As I helped him adjust again, he chuckled. "Why can't I get that?" he asked. Hours later, in the afternoon session, there he was again: impelling himself toward the mat, contracting his neck and shoulders with such force that he was barely able to breathe. I encouraged him to use his body awareness to rediscover the brand-new version of Downward Dog that we'd created together. When the afternoon session ended, he remarked how hard it was to remember the changes. "The old way is incredibly easy to slip into," he said. "It's automatic."

Peter's persistent movement pattern, like all patterns of thought, emotion, and behavior, didn't stem from a lack of desire to change. He knew intellectually that his habitual way of moving caused pain and stress. But just beyond his awareness, his body kept repeating these painful movements. Peter was practicing yoga in a way that reinforced the very patterns he wanted to change. I see this tendency in so many people. It's important to appreciate how long, and in how many ways, we've traced and retraced our mind and body patterns. It's equally important to recognize that with awareness and attention, we can unlearn them.

Our Capacity for Change

Given their irresistible magnetism and the stealth with which they attract and wire in new experiences, can we really learn to rewire our patterns? The answer is *yes*. We *can* rewire the mind and the body. Neuroscientists have a lot to say about this rewiring, which is called *neuroplasticity*. Neuroplasticity refers to the brain's extraordinary capacity to transform with experience. Amazingly, it all goes back to the idea of—you guessed it—repetition. When we commit over time to a pursuit such as yoga, our brains forge new connections, grow new cells, increase cell size, or enhance cell activity, among other things. The brain transforms when we repeatedly practice a skill such as playing the piano or hitting a baseball. It also builds patterns through yoga's therapeutic tools: in particular, breath, relaxation, meditation, and postures. We can't avoid repetition; the way we use it, however, is critical. We can take a positive tool (such as deeper breathing) and practice it over and over again to create positive emotional patterns.

What Makes Anxiety and Depression So Powerful?

What makes a pattern more powerful is how much practice you put into it. If you played the piano for only a few weeks as a child, the "piano playing" neural networks in your brain will be fairly weak. Play every day for several years, however, and these neural networks will light up your brain with activity.

Thoughts, emotions, body movements, and postural habits work the same way. Through repetition and practice, they help the brain "learn" anxiety and depression. Only one negative thought creates the weakest of neural links. Have that negative thought again and again, and you solidify the neural networks of depression. Anxiety and depression are elegant examples of neuroplasticity, of the way we learn.

Here's how neuroplasticity works on an emotional level: When you think an anxious thought, experience a feeling of depression, or engage in a frenetic or self-defeating behavior, you stimulate corresponding groups of cells in the brain. Each subsequent repetition wires the pattern in more strongly, forming neural support networks. Over time, these networks create a magnetic pull that becomes difficult to resist. Once you've created a newfound anxiety pattern, the next time something goes wrong you're more likely to be filled with worry.

Furthermore, what happens in one area—the mind, brain, nervous system, or body—is echoed in the others. Every time you experience the flutter of adrenaline that signals anxiety in the nervous system or the heavy, quicksand feeling that heralds depression in the body, the other systems in your mind-body network hear and respond in kind. Chronically worried or negative thoughts change your nervous system's chemistry and wiring. This causes physical changes (such as increased heart rate, blood pressure, rate of respiration, and stress hormones). These body states also affect your mind and nervous system, making you more anxious or depressed.

Say that you ask someone out on a date, and he or she turns you down. *I'm such a loser,* you might think to yourself. *Why doesn't he like me?* or *I've got bad luck in relationships.* These aren't simply "innocent thoughts." They become amplified in your mind-body network in much the same way that social rumors operate. The whisper of "loser" (even a mild one) that comes from your mind is overheard. It gets repeated (in a different language) by the emotional regions of the brain (including the nervous system) that speak it aloud. These emotional systems react to the news by upping your fight-flight-freeze response and increasing your stress hormones. By the time this whisper makes it through your emotional systems and into your body, or vice versa, it has grown to a "shout." Every part of the mind-body network knows about it. This contributes to increased muscle tension, lowered immunity, and so on. A negative thought gathers strength as it travels through your mind-body network. So your negative thoughts, however understandable they may be, can heighten anxiety and depression.

Anxiety and depression may have been carefully constructed and reinforced in us, sometimes for decades. So even when we know that change is possible, it's easy to feel as if the deck is stacked against us in the quest for emotional balance. But it helps to understand which elements of the mind-body network contribute most strongly to the neuroplasticity, the wiring in, of our negative emotional patterns. Each of these elements acts as a medium through which we build our emotional patterns:

1. The nervous system
2. The body
3. Practicing old patterns

The mind has earned a reputation as a major contributor to anxiety and depression, and remains a focus of most modes of psychotherapy. But the careful work of psychotherapy is harder to integrate and translate into change when any one of the following conditions are met: the nervous system is hyperaroused, the body either doesn't agree with positive thinking or maintains the postural or movement patterns of anxiety and depression, or we inadvertently practice old patterns. So the nervous system, the body, and the practicing of patterns are primary agents of neuroplasticity. They can engineer emotional balance, and also create healing. We can balance the nervous system, cultivate a deeper relationship with the body, and practice new, healthier patterns. Each of these three elements builds on the one before it, and together, all three help to create emotional health.

1. The Nervous System and Your Electrical Wiring

A great *New Yorker* cartoon shows a man and a woman, yoga mats in hand, emerging from a class at the "Life Spirit Meditation

Center." They look stressed, not at all relaxed. As they're walking away, the man says to his wife, "As far as I can tell, meditation is just worrying minus the content."[1] This insightful comment gets at the very nature of how the mind and nervous system collaborate in creating anxiety and depression. The mind supplies the *content* of worrying: the things you worry about and the stories you tell about your worries. You might think that if you quiet the mind, your worrying will stop. Yet it doesn't often turn out that way. As this cartoon wisely suggests, even when the mind quiets, an underlying distress may remain. It does so because the nervous system stays on high alert underneath it all, while the body practices its old posture and movement patterns.

Your nervous system includes your brain, spinal cord, nerves, and nerve pathways. Your cells communicate electrically, through nerve impulses, and chemically, through chemical messengers. Your nervous system oversees communication among all the cells in your body. It also regulates countless functions such as heart rate, blood pressure, respiration rate, and wakefulness, which all relate to stress. When it comes to your outer environment, the nervous system acts as a sentry. It patrols the outer world for danger or change. In response to a life-threatening event, it initiates a stress response.

Say you're crossing an alley on your way home. Suddenly, someone in a ski mask and dark clothing pulls out a gun and orders you to hand over all your money. Your sympathetic nervous system is your "first responder." It activates your fight-flight-freeze response. Blood immediately flows to your heart, which pounds faster in preparation for battle or flight. Oxygen moves to your muscles and brain, which readies you for self-defense or escape. Your pupils dilate, which improves your visual focus and helps you see the mugger better. Your sweat glands activate as your body temperature increases, which keeps you from overheating. Your brain's stress centers turn on and flood you with adrenaline, helping you face your attacker, flee the scene, or remain frozen in place. Salivation decreases and digestion is suppressed so you can focus on the challenge at hand, which contributes to the dryness in your mouth and the tension in your stomach.

Your nervous system is designed to jump into high gear when something potentially life-threatening happens. When the danger has passed, it quiets the stress response and returns to its baseline. The dramatic reactions of the stress response have positive aspects. They are necessary in response to danger. They're tolerable and even productive when they occur occasionally and temporarily. In anxiety and depression, however, this doesn't happen. Instead, the nervous system behaves like a race car in need of repair. The "accelerator" (emergency response) moves too quickly and too often into overdrive. It does this even when there's no real danger. Then the "brakes" (the part of the brain that signals when danger has passed) don't work well, and can't bring the nervous system back into neutral gear. This makes the overdrive period last longer than needed.

An anxious or depressed nervous system frequently stimulates its stress centers through the clever use of peptides, or, in the words of noted psychoneuroimmunologist Candace Pert, *molecules of emotion*. These peptides trigger a cascade of stress hormones such as cortisol and epinephrine, which increase blood pressure and reduce immunity. The ability to sound the alarm in the face of danger is healthy, even life-preserving. Yet over time and with repetition, this "lifesaving" response takes its toll on you and can become life-threatening. As we'll see in the next chapter, balancing the nervous system requires us to fix the overactive accelerator and underactive brakes. And breathing techniques and Restorative Yoga happen to be excellent ways of doing precisely that.

Emotions Behave Like Stress

Although you might think that intense emotions are not the same as life-or-death situations and stress, to your nervous system they actually are. Your nervous system responds to danger not only in your outer environment but your inner one. This inner environment is made up of your sensations, thoughts, and emotions. Your brain plays a "trick" on you and encodes strong emotions such as anxiety, depression, sadness, and anger as acute stress. For example, it interprets your partner's lateness after a night out—and your resulting anger and fear—in much the same way as a mugger's attack.

Your intense emotional reactions to your mother's lack of understanding, to a lover's unexpected assertion of independence, or to a friend's poor boundaries can all set off an emergency response.

Here's another trick of the brain: although your nervous system was designed long ago to protect you against saber-toothed tigers and incoming poison spears, it doesn't take a real threat to engage it. A *perceived* danger, even an imaginary one, will do. Repeated fantasies of catching your partner cheating, for example, elicit reactions from your brain as intense as if you'd actually caught him or her with someone else. This amps up your stress response. Over time, your fight-flight-freeze response to real danger can generalize to milder situations. It even applies to the kind of danger that occurs exclusively in your head. Although you might think this emergency response is set off only in anxiety, research shows that's not the case. Both anxiety and depression, it turns out, involve a chronically amplified nervous system. In depression, however, the nervous system may be wired more to the "freeze" setting than to fight or flight.

Our modern lifestyle can also push the nervous system into overdrive. Even if we're used to it, the onslaught of information we process on a daily basis can be enough to trigger in many of us a toxic barrage of chemical messengers such as cortisol. The modern-day nervous system has to contend with BlackBerry devices and e-mail, call forwarding and text messaging, beepers and video games. It doesn't differentiate between a woolly mammoth and systems overload, between warring tribes of hunter-gatherers and workplace adversaries. The modern-day nervous system processes today's incessant electronic requests in much the same way as it would the attacks and invasions of prehistoric life. We've just become so used to the constant, overwhelming demands that we no longer consciously recognize them as stress. To us, multisensory overload is a part of normal, everyday life.

Anxiety and depression patterns don't occur only in the mind. They are also encoded in the body and "written" onto the nervous system. Here's the thing: the nervous system controls change. When the nervous system is in overdrive, we experience and therefore repeat anxiety and depression, so change can't happen. Like

Cerberus, the giant guard dog in Greek and Roman mythology, the hyperalert nervous system prevents small changes from getting through, even the ones that psychotherapy works so hard to implement. It also negatively affects the body, and can cause or worsen muscular tension, chronic pain, or physical illnesses. Think back to the last time you were really stressed out: didn't your body absorb and reflect that stress as well? Perhaps you got sick, or developed stomach issues. This connection between your nervous system and your body can also work in a positive way: a balanced nervous system can change patterns in the body, as I learned long ago from one of my first yoga students.

2. The Body Communicates with the Nervous System

I never expected that the brand-new yoga practice of an eighty-year-old man would influence the course of my career, but that's what happened. My dad was a writer, an anthropologist, and a filmmaker. Despite his passion for watching sports or other body-focused activities such as Cirque du Soleil, he was more comfortable—at least, toward the end of his life—in his head than in his body. In his late seventies, he was diagnosed with a rare neurological disorder and secondary leukemia. As he rounded the corner of his eightieth birthday, he showed signs of listlessness and wrote less and less. One day, while visiting, I mentioned something that my ninety-seven-year-old female client had done in a yoga session. This piqued his curiosity, and he asked me to show him a few poses.

My dad's yoga practice was a revelation to me in several ways. Frail at first, he had trouble standing on one leg or getting down to or up from the floor. Within weeks after he started practicing yoga, however, he was sailing down and jumping up again with little difficulty. His mood rapidly improved, and he wrote more often. Perhaps most impressive, however, was something I didn't expect. My preconceived image of elders doing yoga included stiffness and increasingly limited mobility. Yet in stark contrast to what I saw in his contemporaries, my dad developed both strength and flexibility. When he first began yoga, he could draw his knee to his chest; soon, to his ear. Toward the end of his life, he could nearly place his leg behind his head. I scrutinized him session after session to figure it out. Why, when my students in their twenties and thirties struggled in vain to increase the range of motion in their hips or shoulders, did my father grow more flexible daily? It became a running joke between us: I'd ask him what performance-enhancing drugs he was taking, while he'd laugh happily and refuse to tell me.

Eventually, I came to connect my dad's progress with my understanding of how relaxation affects the nervous system—and how the nervous system in turn influences the body. The nervous system's fight-flight-freeze response causes muscular tension. Due partly to his neurological issues and partly to his yoga practice, his nervous system was rarely, if ever, in overdrive. So his muscles held little tension; naturally, this helped increase his flexibility.

I've seen this connection between the body and the nervous system work the opposite way as well. Olivia, one of my longtime yoga clients and a trauma survivor, has very little flexion, extension, or rotation in her hips. At first, seeing her restricted range of motion, I referred her to an orthopedic doctor. Olivia's MRI scans showed a normal range of motion with no arthritis or skeletal restriction. Yet it was hard for her just to sit on the floor with her legs crossed. The culprit: her hyperalert nervous system maintained the tension in her hips. When Olivia can turn off or regulate this inner alarm, she'll be able to increase her flexibility. Until then, she is focusing on being present with her direct experience of her body.

What does this mean for *our* yoga practice? Certainly, we can use breathing to balance the nervous system. Yet we have another option: because of the feedback loop between the mind, body, and nervous system, we can also use *body relaxation* to calm the nervous system. So we can add the more meditative, relaxing forms of yoga to what we're already practicing. In this way, we address the body directly—and through it, the mind and nervous system.

In trying to balance the nervous system, understanding alone isn't enough. Mental insight, no matter how profound or earth-shattering, turns a light on in the mind but leaves the body in the dark. Change requires new, *embodied* experiences that differ from our customary anxious or depressed ones. Yoga brings us directly into the body. It grounds our insight into experience. Yet a onetime embodied insight isn't enough: We need to *repeat* these embodied experiences of change (a relaxed body, a balanced nervous system) to grow healthier emotional patterns. The trouble is that most of the time, when we're not in the body, we're less present. We're disembodied. We may then unintentionally practice old patterns of anxiety and depression (a tense body, a hyperaroused nervous system) instead.

Recently, at a weekend workshop on yoga for anxiety and depression, I witnessed this principle firsthand. Workshop participants demonstrated in dramatic fashion the contrast between using only the mind, versus the mind *and* body, as a vehicle for growth. First, we went around the room and each person told his story or her personal narrative of anxiety or depression. Story after story of helplessness, self-disgust, chronic fear, and despair emerged. By the time we were halfway through, a cascade of mind-body reactions was in full swing. Nearly every member of the group sagged in defeat: shoulders slumped, eyes downcast, and fidgeting in discomfort. Several dabbed at their eyes with Kleenex. Rather than process what had just happened and perhaps make matters worse, I asked them to move immediately into a therapeutic yoga pose that involved reclining, face-up, back-bending over a block to open the upper thoracic spine and heart area (this resembled the shape of Inversion Pose on page 203). After two minutes or so of deep breathing in the pose, the group members made their way back up to sitting. They looked much more energized and optimistic than they had two minutes earlier. Although I could easily see the striking changes, I asked them to share their experiences. Many practitioners reported with excitement that they felt almost no trace of the hopelessness and depression that had plagued them only minutes before. Several even said that they'd forgotten what we'd been talking about prior to the exercise!

What was the "hidden insight" here? Verbally processing anxiety and depression can actually rehearse and reinforce—in the mind and body—the very experiences we're trying to change. Yet when we bring awareness, breath, and presence *to the body,* and remain there despite pain or discomfort, we can interrupt the negative cycle of anxiety and depression. If I'd shared this insight with my students *verbally,* it would have been hard for them to feel its effects. They needed the *physical* experience of being depressed or anxious, moving into the body, and then emerging without that anxiety and depression, for the insight to be embodied, to be profound and lasting.

3. Patterns That Reinforce Anxiety and Depression

We practice all the time, often without realizing it. Each time we respond to experience with a thought, feeling, movement, action, or self-talk, we rehearse our patterns. For the most part, we're not consciously aware of this rehearsal. Meanwhile, the act of practicing makes our patterns more ingrained and difficult to resist.

Lucy, a young woman in her twenties, came to me at the suggestion of her primary care physician. Lucy wanted help with long-standing depression and acute back pain. She practiced yoga six times per week—*without fail,* she told me. Yet despite her dedication to practice, Lucy still experienced back pain so intense that some days she found it difficult to walk. Her orthopedic doctor recommended that she give up yoga, but she said that was *"not* an option." Lucy couldn't understand why her body was so tight and riddled with pain. Shouldn't she be flexible and pain-free by now? Why weren't things getting better, she wanted to know, when she was doing everything she was supposed to?

Before her second yoga therapy session, Lucy attended one of my public yoga classes, and the answer became clear. She wrestled her body into every pose as though she were trying out for a football team. She breathed shallowly and held her breath so often that she was red in the face. To get her breath back, she was frequently forced to rest (her "least favorite thing") in Child's Pose. Without being aware of it, Lucy held her body so rigid that she couldn't generate any internal relaxation, let alone awareness. She had difficulty adjusting her postures or making modifications. When I assisted her posture in a way that would bring some softening to her body, it felt to me as though her body were rebelling: against me, herself, and even the practice she loved. After the class, Lucy told me she'd been going to a high-octane Power Yoga class daily for two years. "Is that bad for me?" she asked apprehensively. The type of yoga Lucy preferred mattered less than the way she practiced: with the driven energy of a cruel taskmaster who monitored her every move and exacerbated her chronic pain and depression. Unconsciously, Lucy was "repeating" depression in nearly every movement. I see this so often: the mind works hard in psychotherapy or self-study, trying to change our patterns. And all the while, the body and nervous system are steadfastly practicing them.

To rewire our system, we need not strive for perfection. It's enough to aim for healthier patterns. We seek to access and mold our brain's plasticity, its capacity for change. In the process of healing, *practice makes plastic.* Yet as Lucy's experience indicates, your emotional well-being doesn't depend on *whether* you practice yoga, but *what* and *how* you practice. This book is about the *what* and the *how.* An "emotional retraining" manual, it offers you specific new experiences to shift anxiety and depression. As you do the exercises in this chapter and in the rest of part 1, notice how they affect your nervous system and address your body. Feel how they build more awareness of how you think, move, and hold your body in space—and how this relates to your emotional well-being.

Neuroplasticity is encouraging: our brains have the capacity for change. What's more, they constantly respond to new experiences. Neuroplasticity reassures us that we're not condemned to emotional distress for the rest of our lives. It's never too late: my father took up yoga at the age of eighty and changed dramatically because of it. Like him, we have opportunities to shift our emotional patterns throughout our lives. We have a choice, one that we make anew each day. We can allow old experiences to reinforce anxiety and depression, or create new ones that lead to emotional balance. The question is whether we harness the brain's positive capacity for change, or whether we let its negative potential for change harness us.

What are the deep, intrinsic mechanisms that underlie change? As we have just seen, one of this book's central principles is that without changing the nervous system's chronic stress response, engaging the body's participation, and practicing new rather than old patterns, it's almost impossible to access our capacity for change. But before we jump right in to do these things, let's look more closely at neuroplasticity. The better we understand this science of repetition, the more we can use it to our advantage.

Breath Exercise: 1:1 Breathing

In the first breathing exercise (Getting to Know Your Breath, page 28), you observed your breathing patterns and noticed any difference in the length of your inhale and exhale. If you haven't tried Getting to Know Your Breath yet, do so first before moving on to this one, unless you've had a lot of practice with yogic breathing exercises.

In this exercise, 1:1 Breathing, you will begin to regulate your breath. Specifically, you'll equalize the length of your inhale and exhale. As you move into more structured breathwork, make sure that each breathing ratio feels comfortable to you. Discomfort can cause anxiety, which constricts your breath further. If this happens, return to Getting to Know Your Breath. Practice it as many times as possible, and then come back to this exercise.

Get Your Baseline

Before beginning, return to your notes from Getting to Know Your Breath to see whether your inhale or your exhale was longer. This will be your baseline, and tell you which element of your breath to focus on. If your customary breath ratio involves a shorter inhale, you'll focus on lengthening it. Conversely, if your regular breath ratio has a shorter exhale, you'll work on making your exhale longer. Now take a moment to assess your current mental and emotional baseline. Does your mind feel calm? Or are your thoughts fast, racing, and worried?

Do the Practice

Slowly close your eyes and let them relax. Allow the closing of your eyes to signal to your mind, brain, and body that you are moving from outer awareness to inner awareness.

Begin to focus on your breath. Breathe in and out through your nose naturally. The act of noticing in a neutral way—not in a self-improvement kind of way—is important when working with any pattern, be it a breath-related, mental, or emotional pattern. So, observe your breath without trying to change it. While you breathe, count the length of your inhale and exhale. Notice how many counts it takes to breathe in and breathe out. Which is longer today, your inhale or your exhale? This is your natural breath ratio for the day. If today's breath ratio is different than it was in Getting to Know Your Breath (see page 28), just make a note of that.

After a few minutes of observing your breath, begin to lengthen both your inhale and your exhale; see whether you can increase them by just one count. If this new length feels comfortable, take it as a sign that you can move on. If you experienced any difficulty with lengthening your breath, stay with your previous ratio for the remainder of this exercise, or until lengthening the breath by one count feels more natural. It's important not to force the breath to do anything; this will tighten your diaphragm and, most likely, your face and neck muscles. The forcing and tension will also stimulate your nervous system.

Now bring your awareness to whichever part of your breath was shorter, your inhale or your exhale. Begin to lengthen it one count at a time (for several rounds at each count), until your inhale and exhale are equal. Be as patient as you can with yourself; it can take concentration and patience to develop 1:1 breathing. If it feels difficult right now, honor that difficulty by returning to your natural inhale and exhale ratio, or the one that feels best today. When approximately five minutes have passed, slowly open your eyes.

Feel the Difference

When you open your eyes, keep them relaxed and "unfocused" for several moments, still directing your awareness inward. Take a moment to feel the difference. Review your mental and emotional baseline so you remember how you felt before the exercise. Now register any changes you feel, so that you have a sense of how your breath affects you. How does your mind feel? If it has slowed down or is calmer, make a note of that. If your mind feels agitated, record that as well. You could also experience a "neutral" feeling: neither calm nor agitated, but somewhere in between. Write down whatever you notice.

If your mind became more agitated or distracted in response to 1:1 Breathing, you could be exerting too much effort to control your breath. Or, your mind could simply be more agitated today. If you try this exercise several times and each time your mind becomes hyperactive, this is important. It's likely an indication that in the long run, 1:2 Breathing may be more effective for you than 1:1 Breathing.

If you can't yet pinpoint a difference, or don't feel anything "big," that's OK. Sometimes it takes more practice to feel the effects of your breath. You're looking for small changes that will grow into bigger ones over time.

Body Exercise: The Five-Minute Body Check-in

In the first body-centered exercise, Distinguishing between Tension and Relaxation (see page 31), you developed your ability to differentiate between muscular tension, which activates the nervous system, and relaxation, which calms the nervous system. In this exercise, you will build further on those skills and bring deeper awareness into your body. The Five-Minute Body Check-in is designed as a building block for the more advanced self-observation practices you'll find later in this book. It begins by noticing the state of your mind and the level of comfort in your body. If you have difficulty when you first start, return to Distinguishing between Tension and Relaxation. Practice it several times, and then try this exercise again.

Get Your Baseline

Practicing this exercise will help you check in with and inhabit your body. If you tend to live in your head rather than your body, or find it difficult to be in your body due to physical or emotional pain, progress slowly through this exercise. You can even try it for just a couple of minutes and then stop, if you like. Find a quiet space where you will not be disturbed for five to ten minutes. Have your journal or notebook and a pen nearby so you can record any observations afterward.

Take a moment to get a mental and physical baseline for how you feel today. For your mental baseline, give yourself a number on a 1–10 scale, with "10" being extremely anxious and "1" being totally tranquil. For your physical baseline, note your body's level of energy. Use your 1–10 scale, with "10" being extremely energized and "1" being as low-energy as you can imagine.

Do the Practice

Sit comfortably with your legs crossed, with several inches of elevation (a bolster, pillows, or blanket) under your sitting bones. Add pillows or blocks under your thighs to support your knees if they feel better with support. Since comfort is important in helping you inhabit your body, you can adopt any modifications necessary. You can extend your legs, prop your back up against a wall, or lie on your back with your knees bent.

All transitions can benefit from awareness, even the transition from having your eyes open to having them closed. Take a moment to look around you and let your eyes take in anything they wish. Then close your eyes slowly and gently. As you've done in each of your breath and body check-ins, let the closing of your eyes be a signal to your mind, your brain, and your body that you're moving from *outer* awareness (of the things you normally focus on outside of you) to a deep, *internal* awareness (of the things you may not be used to attending to inside of you). This transition, when practiced mindfully, helps you relax your body and quiet your nervous system.

As you breathe slowly through your nose, direct your breath to your eyes. Let your eyeballs relax and move inward, dropping toward the center of your body. As you do this, hold the intention to let your outer sight—your observation of things outside of you—transform into inner sight, or your observation of all the things inside of you. Let your ears also draw inward, coming to join your eyes at the very center of your body. In this way, your outer hearing—the things that you listen to outside of you—becomes a deep, internal listening. With this transition, you begin to build a connection to your inner voice, your wisdom and knowledge.

As you continue your nasal breathing, draw your attention inward and focus on your body. Compassionate observation is one of the most powerful tools with which you can change your patterns; just notice, with compassion, whether there is comfort, discomfort, or strong tension in your body. Now pick a part of your body to focus on—say, your shoulders. Patiently direct your breath to that part of your body (your shoulders). Release any judgmental thoughts that may arise about it. As you inhale, imagine that you are drawing in life force, positive energy, and faith. As you exhale, imagine that you are releasing tension, negativity, and doubt. You *can* change your emotional patterns; you're now learning the skills to help you begin the process of doing so.

Continue directing your breath to different parts of your body, in turn, for several minutes. Then let your attention become more general. Note any physical sensations such as hunger, thirst, comfort, lack of ease, energy, or fatigue. Observe what you are noticing without needing to get caught up in it. As you inhale, just observe what you're noticing. As you exhale, simply let it go.

Now focus once more on your breath. As you breathe slowly through your nose, bring awareness to your mind. Notice the thoughts that surface. What is their quality: Are they distracting? Negative? Hopeful? How fast do they come? Just notice, without judgment. If you become preoccupied and obsess over something, notice that, too. You can even use a 1–10 scale for your thoughts, with "10" being racing, "monkey-like" thoughts that come almost faster than you can handle, and "1" being slow, "molasses-like" thinking.

Bring your focus back to your breath; observe your breath to make sure you're breathing through your nose. Breathe in and out through your nose for several inhales and exhales. Next, draw your awareness and your breath to your feelings. Note the tone of your emotional self today: Are you feeling optimistic? Anxious? Sad? Distressed? Just notice, without needing to become attached to what you are noticing. Become aware of what you're focusing on as you inhale. Let it go as you exhale.

You've now traveled into your body, your mind, and your emotional self. Take a few minutes to breathe quietly, still keeping your focus linked to your breath. When you are ready to begin the transition out of your check-in, let your awareness travel a little closer to the surface and become a bit more aware of your surroundings while still retaining your connection to your inner world.

Feel the Difference

Take a moment to check back in with your body, your mind, and your emotional self. Observe any changes or shifts that have occurred. Stay as impartial as you can when noticing these shifts. When you are ready, gently transition your eyes to open. If you wish, note any observations from your Five Minute Body Check-in. Do you feel a difference, however small? Perhaps your depression or anxiety has lessened a bit. Training your attention inward is one of the ways you can interrupt your anxiety or depression pattern. Why? Because focusing inward brings you to a place where you're not anxious or depressed.

Return to your physical, mental, and emotional baseline; allow any difference you feel to register fully. Do you feel more energy in your body? What about your mind—does your mind feel slower or calmer? And emotionally: do you feel more connected to yourself, or perhaps more compassion for yourself? Note any such differences in your journal so that you can see how inhabiting your body affects you over time.

If you don't feel anything different, this may mean that you live more in your head than in your body, which is normal for many people. You'll just need a little more practice with this check-in to feel a change. If you haven't inhabited your body very much, doing so can take many months to get used to. If you continue your practice of compassionate and neutral self-observation, it will get easier.

↶3

How True Healing Happens

RECENTLY, I WORKED ONE-ON-ONE WITH A PROFESSIONAL athlete just prior to the start of his season. If you've ever followed Boston sports, you'll know that even a month before the season begins, the quest for a championship—and the pressure—is on. This particular young player, whom I'll call Ben, had a history of back problems. Each year, just a couple of months into the season, he got injured and had to miss several weeks. This year, his contract was up. He and the team expressed concerns about his physical condition. Ben had already worked with his personal trainer in the off-season on a variety of elements including core body strength, which supports the spine. After a brief functional mobility assessment, I could tell that Ben's external abdominal muscles were strong. However, his deep, intrinsic core muscles were weak. He could do seventy-five crunches without pausing, yet he had trouble holding a simple Plank Pose (which looks like the beginning of a push-up) with healthy alignment. Within seconds, his legs would start to shake and his lower back would collapse toward the floor. Although Ben had worked hard in the off-season, he skipped the basic core poses. Without a strong foundation, he proceeded straight to the advanced exercises, increasing the likelihood of back strain. I recommended that Ben go back to the beginning and focus on building core body strength. The sequence I designed for him included simple poses, the kind anyone can do. But he had to maintain spinal alignment and deep breathing, a challenge that would make each pose more difficult. In a week or two, I assured him, he could graduate to more advanced core body poses using the same alignment principles. Two problems immediately arose. The first: Ben was reluctant to "go backward," to do the "easy stuff." After all, he was a multimillion-dollar athlete, not a novice. The second: his coaches needed to see quick results in speed, strength, and output or they would bench him. Naturally, they couldn't imagine how the easier exercises would produce the rapid results they wanted. With some negotiation on both sides—me, and Ben's ego and coaches—we agreed to use the program I designed for two weeks and then reevaluate. Each day, Ben began at the beginning and progressed through the series. To his surprise, he built true core body strength quickly. Within the two-week trial period, his back pain disappeared and hasn't returned since. He continued to use the careful progressive sequence we designed together. Soon, his daily training session could begin with more challenging core body postures. In a few months, something happened that surprised him: because his core body grew stronger, his peripheral muscles (such as the arms, legs, and upper trunk) didn't need to overcompensate, and they tired less quickly. Three months into the season, when Ben typically fell into a slump or got injured, his statistics, the results everyone wanted, improved in every area. The key part: his power surge didn't come just from repeating intelligent techniques, but also from building them in a progressive sequence, with patience, over time.

The previous chapter focused on repetition, an important part of changing anxiety and depression. Repetition means that practicing is key. But choosing our therapeutic tools wisely and sequencing them well is every bit as important. So *what* do we practice? And how do we sequence our therapeutic tools to create incremental, healthy change?

Incremental Change

Let's take a moment to revisit the concept of instant healing, and see how it applies to change. In most of us, an unconscious battle rages over change. What we want and what we need are at odds.

The mind, or ego, wants instant and measurable results. It likes to tackle the hardest things or the highest level first. However, the rest of us, especially the nervous system, isn't able to assimilate instant transformation. Most of the time, true change can't happen all at once. It needs a foundation, a supportive framework. Just like Ben, we start with small experiences, build on them, and progress over time. This isn't bad news but for many of us, impatient with the slow, steady progress that growth requires, it can certainly feel that way. I've experienced the same impatience and desire for instant results myself.

When I first began to do yoga, more than eighteen years ago, I was very taken with its physical aspects. One posture in particular captured my attention: Forearm Balancing Pose. In this pose, you balance on just your forearms and extend your legs straight up in the air: like a headstand, only on the forearms. As a beginner, I had no idea how to do the pose or what its different components were. Nevertheless, my teachers thought I should do it, and my ego agreed. So I repeatedly pushed myself to get into it; each time, I'd fall out of the pose sideways. Unable to control my descent, I'd invariably turn my head to the side and get rug burns high on my cheekbones, right at my eye sockets. For many weeks, I walked around with angry red abrasions where I'd fallen, looking like ballplayers who wear pitch under their eyes to deflect the sun. One day, it occurred to me that pushing for the pose made me miserable. I decided not to try it for six months. I practiced foundational yoga poses every day and began to generate more intelligence in my body. I reflected on which poses and what actions were necessary for getting into Forearm Balancing Pose: openness in the shoulders, core body strength, leg strength, arm strength, and a large dose of fearlessness. Day after day, I practiced and integrated these necessary components. I could feel myself inching closer to the pose every day, but resisted trying again too soon. I found sweetness in the simple building of awareness in my body. One day, I knew without a doubt that each element of the pose had ripened, and the pose was waiting for me to try again. With a combination of excitement, and not a little regret for leaving this stage behind, I paused at the moment in my practice where the pose would come. I inhaled. I exhaled and kicked up.

I stayed, breathing deeply and tasting the pose, for over one minute. My lesson: a mindful foundation helps us integrate growth more smoothly. In other words, steady and progressive change is the kind that lasts. If I told you that I learned this lesson that day and never forgot it, that wouldn't be the truth. I've had to learn and relearn it over and over again in many aspects of my life.

We can't accomplish something that's too far outside the limits of our capabilities without help of some kind. There's a technical term for this: the *zone of proximal development.*[1] While you don't need to know the educational theory behind it, the concept is important. It means we can't go from point A to point Z (say, from extreme anxiety to total calm) in one fell swoop the way we might like to. The brain best accommodates smaller increments of change with certain kinds of help (such as therapeutic yoga). Progressing from point A to point C or D, for instance (say, from extreme anxiety to just a strong sense of worry), supports integration and change. This means that the desire for immediate results (and instant healing) isn't just a harmless fantasy. In real life it's next to impossible, aggravates the nervous system, and adds unnecessary pressure when we're trying to change our patterns.

Why is this lesson so hard for us to learn? The mind often mistrusts the body. It thinks of the body as primitive. The mind likes to do things faster, better, perfectly—right away. It often tries to "help" that happen by overriding the body's intelligence and its natural sense of what it can and can't do. In the physical practice of yoga, or *asana,* we need to develop the basic foundations for difficult postures, as I had to do in order to balance on my forearms. Without that development, we risk forcing the body to do something before it is ready. This poses a dilemma: if we don't strive to "get there" instantly, we can feel disappointed. Yet if we do force the body, we face consequences. First, the changes we make don't fully integrate into our lives. Second, when using force, we "practice" internal pressure and lack of compassion. In both cases, we end up with the inner harm or self-judgment that characterizes anxiety and depression.

So how does all this relate to emotional balance? Think of yoga's physically demanding, or "crescendo," poses as similar to emotionally charged situations. For these crescendo poses to be successful, they require several smaller components. As we've discussed, to get into and out of forearm balance, you need shoulder flexibility, core strength, arm and leg strength, balancing ability, and the capacity to try new things. Emotional balance works in much the same way. Say that you need to confront an emotionally distant partner. Let's break this situation down into its parts, like we did for Forearm Balancing Pose. There are several elements: first, you would feel the feelings of hurt and anger toward your partner without letting them consume you. Second, you would recover from the hurt and anger afterward. Third, you'd also want to separate the outcome—whether your spouse changes his or her behavior—from your sense of self-worth. To do all this, though, takes time and effort. You wouldn't expect to engineer a mature confrontation, manage its aftereffects, and then let go of the outcome right away. Ideally, you'd first spend time learning to inhabit your body fully and noticing the difference between activation *and* calm. You would then practice breathing through and being present with difficult emotions. You would learn how to calm the nervous system and make it less reactive to your partner's coldness or withdrawal. This would give you the ability to manage your physiological reactions to emotion. You'd want to practice all this when things are already going smoothly. Then you could put your abilities to use in more challenging situations, working up gradually to the interaction with your spouse. This is how you develop change progressively, in a truly integrative way, rather than expecting it to come all at once. So in order to build this type of progressive and integrative change, what kind of experiences do you need? A hint: they're not the dramatic ones you may have come to expect.

The Power of Subtle Practices

When we suffer from anxiety or depression, we can be goal-oriented; we naturally want to feel better right away. And the people who care about us also want us to improve as quickly as possible. So we may push for the more dramatic methods of healing: the advanced pose, the intense yoga workout, the marathon meditation. Yet focusing on immediate results places more value on the final *goal* of being healed than on the process of getting there. When we push for immediate results and instant healing, we never inhabit the important in-between phase, which is where much of the learning and growth actually happen. As we'll see in chapter 5, this in-between phase is important in healing anxiety and depression.

When I teach workshops on emotional health, participants often expect a "yogic prescription." They want several poses they can do for anxiety or depression. This expectation isn't unusual; I encounter it in conference settings, magazine interviews, even television segments. In the last year alone, colleagues and writers have asked me for three simple poses or yogic techniques to help with anxiety, depression, insomnia, seasonal affective disorder, career transitions, and improving the way we manage time. And just the other day on the Internet, I saw the headline "Yoga Pose to Improve Your Sex Life." It's natural to want a recipe for quick interventions that will help us feel better right away. And as research has shown, yoga's physical postures do improve anxiety and depression. Yet when it comes to emotional health, it's not that simple. What counts are not the poses that we do, but the way we gradually build awareness *within* the postures and the mindfulness we bring to them. For instance, we can do a physically powerful pose with very little presence or awareness and not see much change. Or we can inhabit the subtlest of postures or practice the most elementary breathing technique with awareness and see great benefit over time. In every workshop, I try to give people a firsthand experience of this.

When I teach yoga for anxiety and depression, I begin by explaining what gets in the way of change, how change really happens, and the importance of repeating subtle interventions in a progressive sequence over time. To help people embody this understanding, I introduce over twenty interventions or tools. Each time they practice one, I ask people to do a brief mind and body check-in to get their "before" picture or baseline. Then, they practice the exercise. Right away, they do a new check-in to get their "after" picture and compare it with their baseline. This allows them to feel and evaluate how helpful the exercise has been for them. Then, I put the exercise into a therapeutic context. I explain how to use each therapeutic tool on its own, group it with others in a cohesive practice, or integrate it into an already established yoga practice. I remind them that they also (as in the case of the neck and throat adjustment that you'll find at the end of this chapter) want to practice these tools in their lives off the mat, such as at their desk, in the car, or while working out. Then, at the end of the workshop, we review each of the interventions we've used. You might think that this careful process would give people a clear menu of practices for changing their emotional patterns, but it doesn't always work that way.

Even after hearing about the power of subtle tools, they can "default" to their original concept of how change happens. At the end of one workshop, for instance, after trying the method above with twenty-four exercises, a participant surprised me by saying that she'd been given "no tools" to address her emotional patterns. And many others respond to the subtle practices of therapeutic yoga by asking for "more yoga." They expect to sweat, to be challenged physically in a discrete, time-limited, 30- to 90-minute yoga practice with a beginning and an end, in order to feel better emotionally. Our cultural conditioning toward big changes and instant results can cause many of us to overlook the power of these subtle practices. When I introduce a subtle therapeutic tool in a workshop, I always watch for reaction; at times, people can seem a little disappointed. *"This is it?"* They sometimes ask. "What does this have to do with anxiety and depression?" They don't want "baby" poses such as the core body poses that I gave Ben, the athlete you met at the beginning of this chapter.

At first it surprised me that the subtler, less physically active practices such as breathwork, postural adjustments, and Restorative Yoga don't feel to some people like *real* yoga. But it makes sense when we consider it in light of the "instant makeover" culture in which we live. Seeing this preference for "intense" or prescriptive practices has taught me something: in the process of developing emotional balance, most of us start first with "gross" (basic) awareness. We begin our journey to emotional balance by understanding how *big* things in our lives (the loss of a job, a new relationship, or a fight with a loved one, for example) contribute to anxiety and depression. We expect equally big tools (challenging poses, sweat-inducing or intense physical practices, or emotionally-charged breakthroughs) to heal them. Yet we make a key mistake in thinking that only dramatic experiences, negative or positive, create or heal anxiety and depression.

Yoga's more subtle tools (breathing exercises, focused awareness, postural alignment work, and restorative postures) are powerful. They challenge our "instant healing" programming. They provide us with the assistance we need to develop our awareness in small, easier-to-assimilate steps. In educational theory, this is called *scaffolding*. When we practice them mindfully, these subtle tools become a sustainable practice that we can adjust, refine, and rely on for the rest of our lives. Recently, a man in one of my workshops responded to the concept of a lifelong practice with distress, saying, "Do I really have to do this for the rest of my life just to feel better?"

These therapeutic tools are not, as this man feared, some sort of therapeutic "life sentence." They're not prescriptions that need to be taken, tasks that must be performed, or another set of self-improvement techniques. Rather, this dynamic, alive set of tools offers you a *sustainable therapeutic practice*. Through your relationship with these tools and with your mind and body, you can adapt to your changing needs over the course of a lifetime. If you wish, you can use these subtle tools as a companion to the dramatic ones, to the active practices you already do. But don't overlook these subtle practices for what they are: a direct path to optimal emotional functioning.

Here's an example of how a subtle therapeutic tool might hold surprising benefits for you. In most of my workshops, I teach participants the neck and throat adjustment at the end of this chapter (Going Up the Stairs Backward, page 75). I let them know in advance that this subtle adjustment can be difficult to sense, and that they might have to try it ten times before they feel its effects. Before teaching people the adjustment, I frequently ask them to assume their natural, everyday seated posture and get their baseline levels of mental agitation and physical energy. Many report feeling tired and unmotivated. Their physical energy might be low (depressed body), high (anxious body), or somewhere in the middle. Their thoughts may be either slow (depressed mind), racing (anxious mind), or somewhere in between. We then go through the technique, which is designed to free up space at the front of the throat, align the cervical spine, and enhance breathing—all factors which help balance the mind and nervous system. Afterward, I ask them to note the level of energy in their bodies and the speed of their thoughts. Nearly all of them report increased physical energy and greater mental calm or focus. Some even mention a sense of "lightness" and "balanced mental alertness." They're understandably amazed to find that such a seemingly simple adjustment can bring about so much change. Then, we discuss how many instances there are off the mat in which this head and neck adjustment becomes significant: working at a desk, driving, making dinner, or waiting in line at the bank. Even so, it can still be hard to change the bias we have against subtle work; only hours after experiencing the transformative effects of this exercise, some people ask, "Can you tell us again why you taught that thing with the throat?" Even after we've experienced the benefit of these subtle tools, we may still have to combat our long-standing paradigm of healing, which accords importance mainly to dramatic interventions.

It takes time, practice, and awareness to change our preconceived image of how healing happens. Tina, a workshop participant who'd been skeptical about this adjustment, shared her experience with the group at the end of one weekend. She did the neck and throat adjustment on the first day and didn't feel a thing. She went home and tried it on her husband and her children. She saw how it changed their posture and affected their mood. She tried it again on herself and didn't feel any different. Only on the last day of the workshop, when Tina felt someone else assist her, did it begin to make sense. She could feel the adjustment change her body, and could register its mood-enhancing benefits. Tina finally experienced how powerful a seemingly insignificant exercise can be. But it took repetition, several different ways of trying, and a good deal of patience for her to get there. Once she got it, she began to practice it outside of yoga class, helping to spread its mood-enhancing benefits.

Perhaps at times we feel that things are so hopeless, it would take a miracle to change them. We may believe that subtle practices such as breathing and relaxation can't possibly stand up to the bewitching power of anxiety and depression. But this belief flies in the face of what neuroscience has proved about how we learn: neural networks are formed through the ongoing repetition and *progressive building* of new thoughts, emotions, and behaviors. What's more, the nervous system responds with great sensitivity to slight changes in our inner and outer environments. Large-scale or dramatic changes often stimulate the same emergency response system that, as we learned in chapter 2, strengthens the patterns of anxiety and depression. No matter how much we may yearn for them, these dramatic changes "freak out" the nervous system. In contrast, yoga's subtle practices help keep the nervous system balanced. They ensure better, more solid integration of new experiences. Seemingly minor thoughts, shifts in degrees of nervous system relaxation, changes in breath ratios or depth, adjustments in our ability to be present, and refinements in our postural and movement patterns all contribute to either emotional imbalance or emotional well-being. They reduce our tendency to backslide into anxiety and depression when things get difficult. As in the old fable of the tortoise and the hare, when it comes to emotional balance, slow and steady wins the race.

Change Can Happen Silently

As we practice these small interventions, improvement can occur against a backdrop of disbelief—of feeling as if nothing is working. This is because there's a delay between what the brain is already doing and what we consciously register. We can be doing a subtle practice and experiencing a positive effect, and just not yet know it. To illustrate, take the way we respond to danger. Just as the emotional regions of the brain encode "danger" immediately, they also register that the danger has passed. All this may happen before we're consciously aware of it. Likewise, when it comes to changing our emotional patterns, we can move into a healthier pattern on deeper, less conscious levels long before we register awareness of the change.

This happens even on a physical level. Jane, a student of mine, experienced this delay when she traveled to Asia for a year to study architecture. She did very little yoga practice while she was there. But because people in Asia often talk and eat in a squatting position, she did a lot of squatting. She returned with much more openness in her hips than she'd ever had. But her "new" yoga practice looked just like the old one: she guarded her body in hip openers, not deepening into the poses the way she now could. During a private yoga session, when I commented on the sudden openness in her hips, Jane was astonished. With guidance, she was able to embody this new openness and get into postures she couldn't previously access. She just needed time to become aware of the change and integrate it into her practice.

Imagine how this delay might affect you if you're trying a new tool to lift depression. You might regulate your breath, do a Restorative Yoga sequence, or practice active postures. All the while, your brain forges new neural connections. Because these connections take a while to reach your conscious awareness, you may feel as if nothing new is happening. David, a yoga therapy client, was plagued by a mixture of depression and anxiety. He felt so drained just getting through a day's work that he parked himself on the couch all night, and he hadn't attended any of his son's youth hockey games for a year. On the other hand, David's mind was always hyperactive and worried, imagining frightening scenarios such as his son being injured. After several months of yoga therapy, which included breathwork, Sun Salutations, and restorative postures, David's mind became calmer and quieter. He criticized his wife much less, and made important gains in self-compassion. Yet David remained so preoccupied with his low energy level and his inability to go to social gatherings that he had difficulty seeing all the positive gains he'd made. It wasn't until he found himself cheering at his son's playoff game that David realized how far he'd come. In time, he realized that changes were actually taking place just beyond his awareness, and that he could trust the process. Understanding the need for gradual, progressive change, the importance of incremental healing, and the delay between *actual* change and *felt* change can help you stick with these subtle, healing practices, even if you're not yet sure they're working.

Thinking about how change really happens, how true and lasting healing occurs, can give us hope. Our negative patterns were wired into us bit by bit over a long period of time. And that's how they transform: with determination, a little bit at a time, over the long haul. This may at first seem frustrating; why should change take so long? But when we think about how much time we've spent setting our patterns in place, it's not that long at all. John Farrell, the pitching coach for the Boston Red Sox, recently wove Eastern philosophy into an inspirational talk he gave to his players. "Your work in getting to know your own body," he told the guys, "is never done." The same is true of our journey toward emotional balance. Using subtle interventions, we "work" on ourselves over time. But there's no endpoint to reach; the work is just a process that we engage in on an ongoing basis. The good news is that when our awareness reaches a critical level, it gains momentum.

How Therapeutic Yoga Creates a Foundation for Change

The subtle interventions of therapeutic yoga also help bypass the verbal processing that can get in the way of change. Lauren, a forty-four-year-old yoga therapy client, discovered the power of body-focused therapeutic work in one of her sessions. Lauren worked as a trader in a high-intensity investment firm. She found it hard to turn down the volume on her stress at the end of the day, so I often saw her in high-stress mode: talking fast, physically agitated, fidgety, and jumping from one topic to the next. The way her boss made her perform menial tasks, her secretary's too-long lunch breaks, and her coworkers' backstabbing business ethics all evoked intense emotion. Lauren usually felt the urge to update me on all these happenings before we started. As a result, the updates often swallowed up the bulk of her sessions. Recently, following a confrontation with a fellow trader, she began a session highly agitated. I suggested we skip the update, go straight to the yoga, breathe, and let her be in her body—all interventions that had helped so much in past sessions. Yet Lauren resisted. She wanted to "talk it out" for a minute or two, convinced it would help her feel better. As we talked in the easy chairs in front of her fireplace, one minute stretched into two, then five, then ten. Her voice rose by several decibels. She began to punctuate her story with wild swings of her arm. Her breathing grew more shallow and rapid. Lauren's emotions heightened rather than calmed. Several times, I suggested that we begin the practice, but she demurred. Finally, her tirade came to a halt. She felt even worse than before she'd started talking, and reasoned that maybe a little yoga could help. Lauren came to her mat and breathed. Then we began some simple Sun Salutations. Within several minutes of deep breathing linked with simple movement, things changed. Lauren's voice quieted. Her thoughts slowed. Her breathing became more even. Her anger softened. "Why didn't we do this twenty minutes ago?" she asked laughingly. We agreed that the next time she got worked up, we'd fast-forward through the talking part and proceed directly to yoga.

What does this powerful, body-centered form of yoga therapy mean for talk therapy? First, we can give credit where it's due. Psychotherapy has revolutionized the treatment of emotional illness and pain. In my father's lifetime, talking about one's personal problems was taboo. People were expected to bear the burden of emotional illness and pain silently and stoically. Yet since the mid-1980s, psychotherapy has been a medium for people to express and understand suffering. Options are now so diversified that you can choose from a large menu of therapies: cognitive, cognitive-behavioral, mindfulness-based, internal family systems, and many more. One of psychotherapy's most important contributions to healing has been the provision of a safe place for people to share their story with a compassionate, experienced listener. Giving voice to deep emotional pain and trauma releases many people from an inner prison of silence. Having that story not judged, but received with compassion, can ignite the process of healing.

In some cases, however, we've become conditioned to processing our emotions mentally and verbally. We do it with friends, family, coworkers, even the people in line next to us at the grocery store. We do it with ourselves, internally and out loud. But for people with anxiety and depression, telling these stories can cross the line from therapeutic to negative and repetitive—a form of neuroplasticity that makes painful emotional patterns worse. Many times in my psychotherapy practice, a client would ask, "Don't you get bored having to listen to the same old story every week?" People often recognize that even though the setting or characters may change, their story pops up repeatedly. It's not a matter of boredom for psychotherapists. It's that stories require us to perform a difficult balancing act: they have to negotiate the precarious tightrope walk between listening therapeutically and not encouraging the same old story to come up again and again, which signals the mind-body network that anxiety and depression are still alive.

My experience with Lauren (and many others) showed me something important: mental and verbal processing can cause us to *rehearse* negative emotional patterns. This contributes to nervous system arousal, as it did for Lauren, and slows the progress of emotional change. It's not that we shouldn't process at all, of course. But we can help the mind to quiet. And we can involve the body in processing. This accelerates therapy—it can even, as we'll see in the next chapter, begin to change the nature of our stories.

Mind-Body Therapy: A New Model for Healing Emotional Pain

Can we really continue to leave the body out of the healing process? The effectiveness of yoga therapy challenges our current model of healing through mental and verbal processing. At many venues where I teach, the psychotherapists in attendance have begun to train in yoga, to integrate the body into psychotherapy. Some already use methods such as EMDR (eye movement desensitization and reprocessing) to calm the nervous system. So where then does processing fit in? And can we process *through* the body instead of around it?

Take the treatment of trauma, as an example. Trauma has roots not just in the mind, but also in the body. Pain can be trapped in the body in a way that the mind can't easily reach, let alone discharge. Trauma survivors can progress fairly well in therapy in terms of conceptual understanding. They can recognize the cause of their fears and learn not to be immobilized by them. Yet they can still experience cycles of panic and crippling anxiety, which alternate with despondency and deep depression. Often, they feel trapped inside their bodies. Recognizing this, trauma specialists have begun to integrate breathwork, meditation, and gentle yoga-based movement into their treatment plans. For people who have experienced trauma, a carefully designed and gentle active yoga practice can help release inner tension and agitation. It can also prepare practitioners for any discomfort that might arise in the stillness of restorative postures, enabling them to relax more deeply and balance their nervous systems.

Ariana, one of my students, is a trauma survivor. For the first year of her active yoga practice, she seemed at war with her body. Like many people with post-traumatic stress disorder (PTSD), she alternated between intense physical and mental anxiety, and acute physical and mental depression. In active yoga classes, she'd expend all her energy early on. In some postures, such as Upward Dog, she would force her body to bend so deeply and with such intensity that her neck and jaw muscles clenched with tension. At times, with an almost military determination, she'd order her body into positions it wasn't ready to handle. In several instances, she injured her wrists trying to get into Crow Pose, an arm-balancing posture. Late in the class she'd collapse, sprawled on her mat in no particular pose at all, muttering under her breath. The few words I could catch always berated her body for what it couldn't yet do. When it came to Restorative Yoga, the stillness felt nearly intolerable to Ariana. This wasn't only because her mind remained active, but because the memories and sensations stored in her body hammered at the door of her awareness, trying hard to get out. Ariana could spend only five minutes in a restorative posture before needing to worry incessantly at her props, get up, or pace the room. We could have talked about these issues verbally, but I wondered what that would accomplish; she'd already processed them at length in psychotherapy.

To address her extremes of agitation and lethargy, I tried something different. When Ariana was in "sergeant mode," I gave her a bolster so she could try Supported Child's Pose for a minute or so instead. And when she entered "surrender mode," I'd pass close by and encourage her to deepen her audible Ujjayi breath, a breathing technique used in Vinyasa Yoga. She'd make an occasional joke about the "war zone" her body entered in class; I'd offer gentle encouragement and we'd continue. After a few months, I noticed that Ariana got her own bolster and did Supported Child's Pose throughout the class whenever she needed. She pushed less hard in each pose; her body held less tension and could therefore enter postures with greater ease. Her energy levels remained more consistent, and I no longer saw her collapse on her mat in frustration. Ariana became exhilarated by a new friendliness toward her body. "My body and I have begun peace talks!" she told me one day. I could see this, too; she began to accept modifications for poses rather than forcing her body into them. In Restorative Yoga, Ariana made a great breakthrough when she finally learned to experience and breathe through her body's pain and anger. She found that over time, the simple acts of breathing, awareness, and relaxation helped her stay with her direct experience of her body. Her sense of humor emerged, and she seemed to enjoy class more. She grew better able to endure the intense internal pressure and residue of trauma, and to realize that they could pass.

In addition to my Restorative Yoga classes, I teach active Vinyasa Yoga classes that integrate breath with movement. Unlike typical Power Yoga or Vinyasa Yoga classes, however, the movement between poses is very slow. This allows less time for escape or dissociation, and makes the practice more physically and mentally challenging. Yet the slowness provides too much time for us to simply fall into rote movement patterns. We can approach the precipice of tight places, restriction, physical difficulty, or emotional turmoil, and bring our breath to these junctures.

When new students come to class, I see and appreciate how hard it is for them to be present when the body and inner self are so vulnerable, so exposed. I feel that vulnerability right along with them. Eventually, if they stick with the practice, something beautiful happens. At some point, weeks or months along, a sudden shift occurs. They become more present with their body and mind. Tight parts of the body begin to open and create space. Alignment improves. They seem connected internally, and energy just flows better. This moment is not an esoteric, hard-to-define thing: they can feel it as much as I can witness it. You'll be able to feel it, too: that critical place where the repetition and sequence of the tools you try, and the awareness they generate, reach their emotional "tipping point." From that point on, though we still need to nourish it, awareness is more self-generating and self-sustaining.

We need not give up processing entirely. We can continue to tell stories mindfully, with awareness. We can sense when they've reached the limits of their usefulness and crossed over into a rehearsal of negative thought patterns. Through yoga, we can also give the body room to work its way through our mental insights, to process in its own time and rhythm.

A psychiatrist colleague recently marveled to me at the difference he saw between the yoga practitioners and nonpractitioners who came to him for help. In every case, he said, yoga practitioners seeking help for anxiety and depression were better able to communicate about their pain. They could differentiate between symptoms in the body and in the mind. They could describe internal sensations with greater accuracy. His clients' self-awareness helped him to be a better physician. It made accurate diagnosis and treatment much easier.

Yogic methods that calm the nervous system, address the body, and change *how* we process can be integrated directly into a psychotherapy session. Recently, a social worker who refers clients to our yoga therapy center sent me an e-mail saying, "I don't know what this stuff is about or why it works. All I can say is, the part of our sessions that involves Restorative Yoga is deeper and more powerful."

The yoga therapy tools featured in this book are meditative. Neuroscientists have generated a growing body of research on the benefits of meditation for the brain and, in particular, for emotional health. Partly because of this, some psychotherapists now integrate Buddhist principles and mindfulness techniques into their work with clients. Buddhism and mindfulness-based awareness train the mind to observe itself with detachment and to be a compassionate, impartial witness to direct experience. Here's how this applies to psychotherapy: First, the therapist models this detached (but not uncaring) observation. Next, the client internalizes it. The mind then develops an ability to compassionately witness itself in the midst of emotional turmoil.

Therapeutic yoga takes this training one step further. It helps create a foundational framework for internal awareness. It does this not just through the mind, the "thinker," but also through the body, the "breather." By bringing direct experience into the body, we feel the ebb and flow of mental life and the fluctuations of physical existence *at the same time.* We help the mind learn to be, rather than simply to think.

Yoga is an extraordinary method of mind-body medicine. In the next chapter, we'll explore five *specific* elements of yoga that help build new patterns. You can integrate these techniques into your life, or your current forms of treatment, as soon as you like.

⌒ Breath Exercise: 1:2 Breathing

In the first breathing exercise, Getting to Know Your Breath (page 28), you observed your natural breathing ratio (the relationship between the length of your inhale and exhale). In the second, 1:1 Breathing (page 48), you began to regulate your breath, matching your inhale to your exhale. If 1:1 Breathing was uncomfortable for you in any way, consider returning to Getting to Know Your Breath and practicing it several times. Then progress to 1:1 Breathing; stay with it until you reach a better level of comfort before moving on.

In this exercise, 1:2 Breathing, you'll deliberately make your exhale twice as long as your inhale. This breath ratio slows your heart rate and calms your nervous system, making it one of your most powerful tools for emotional balance. Note that this exercise asks you to *gradually*, rather than *immediately*, make your exhale double the length of your inhale. This is because the 1:2 inhale-to-exhale ratio can be difficult, especially for people with anxiety. Gradually lengthening the exhale helps you work up to a 1:2 ratio slowly. It also enables you to notice right away if discomfort occurs when you try to make your exhale longer. At first, you may feel as though you don't have enough oxygen for the longer exhale. If this happens, or you experience discomfort at any point, return to the last exhale length with which you felt comfortable. Alternatively, practice 1:1 Breathing instead.

Get Your Baseline

Before beginning, take your mental and emotional baseline: How is your mind functioning now? Are your thoughts slow and sluggish, and/or focused on the past? Are they racing, worried, and/or focused on the future? Or are they balanced between these two extremes? Record your mental baseline before beginning.

If you would like to test the rapid effects of 1:2 Breathing (or a longer exhale) on your heart rate, take your pulse for sixty seconds, either on your wrist or on your neck, before beginning. Write down your current number of beats per minute. Make sure that you're not doing this exercise directly after awakening from sleep, when your heart rate would normally be much lower than usual.

Do the Practice

Slowly close your eyes. Breathe through your nose. Direct your neutral, compassionate observation to your breath. As you breathe, count the length of your inhale and your exhale; you can use about one second for each count, if you wish. Do this for two to five minutes, or for a length of time that is comfortable for you.

Now begin to lengthen both your inhale and your exhale. See if you can increase each by a couple of counts, or approximate seconds. When your breath is longer but still stable, experiment by lengthening the exhale. At first, make it just one count longer than your inhale. For instance, if you breathe in for two counts, let your exhale be three counts. If you breathe in for three counts, let your exhale be four counts, and so on. See how the longer exhale feels.

If your breathing remains comfortable here, transition to an even longer exhale; make your exhale two counts longer than your inhale. Try not to move out of your comfort range. Signs of discomfort might include trouble breathing or anxiety about being able to breathe in again or exhale fully. Anytime you feel uncomfortable, return to the last breath ratio that felt good to you.

If exhaling for two counts longer than your inhale is comfortable, you can experiment with 1:2 Breathing. Slowly increase the length of your exhale until it is twice the count of your inhale. If you breathe in for two counts, exhale for four; if you breathe in for three counts, exhale for six; and so on. Do this practice for about three to five minutes.

Feel the Difference

Slowly open your eyes. If you wish to measure the impact of the double-length exhale on your heart rate, take your pulse for sixty seconds and write it down. Note the difference between your pulse before you started this exercise and your present pulse. If it doesn't drop, note that too. It's common for the pulse to drop, sometimes significantly, as a result of this exercise.

Now bring your attention to your mind. Have your thoughts become slower or calmer? What about your emotions: Do they feel more balanced or even-keeled than before? And your body: Is it more relaxed? Note any changes in your journal, so you can see how these changes build and grow over time and with consistent practice. Remember that due to the delay between change and awareness of change (discussed earlier in this chapter), it's possible for your pulse to drop but for you not to feel any mental difference just yet. If this is the case, don't be concerned. As you practice awareness-generating techniques, you'll start to feel the difference sooner.

However, if you've repeated this exercise many times and your mind, body, and emotions feel no different, perhaps you've moved on to 1:2 Breathing too soon. Try practicing Getting to Know Your Breath (page 28) and 1:1 Breathing (page 48) again several times and then come back to this exercise. Remember, although breathing seems as if it should be easy, regulated breathing can be difficult. Allowing yourself time to progress through these exercises gradually will ensure that the benefits take root in your nervous system, and make it more likely that you'll enjoy breathwork.

Body Exercise: Going Up the Stairs Backward

The first two body-centered exercises in this book, Distinguishing between Tension and Relaxation and the Five-Minute Body Check-in, helped you refine your body awareness. These exercises also deepened your perception of physical comfort (which relaxes your nervous system) and discomfort (which can activate your nervous system). These exercises are preludes to the Restorative Yoga practice. If either exercise felt difficult or unnatural to you, consider spending more time with them before moving on to this one. Going Up the Stairs Backward is a postural alignment exercise designed to open your neck and throat area, deepen your breath, and lift your mood. If you find it difficult to know whether you're doing it right, observe yourself from the side using a mirror. You can also ask someone to watch you and tell you if he or she can see a difference in your head and neck alignment.

Get Your Baseline

Before practicing this exercise, assume a comfortable seated position with elevation under your sitting bones. Allow yourself to assume your normal, everyday spinal alignment rather than feeling you need to sit up straight. Then take a minute with your eyes closed to check in with your body. How much physical energy do you feel? Is your body "amped up" with high energy? Tired and lethargic? Or somewhere in between? Make a note of this. Then let your awareness move into your mind. Notice the speed at which your thoughts are flowing: Are they fast, medium, or slow? Record the baselines you obtained in your body and mind: your "before" picture. Soon, you will compare them to how you feel following the exercise: your "after" picture.

Do the Practice

If this is your first time adjusting your own alignment, you may feel a little strange doing so. Just approach this experience with a spirit of exploration, and give yourself some time. Remember that your neck and throat are sensitive; your touch should feel gentle, with very little pressure. Practice this postural adjustment in one of two ways: with your back against a wall or at a side angle to a mirror. You can be seated, with a blanket under you for support, or standing. If you don't have a full-length mirror, standing will help you see yourself better.

As you sit or stand, breathe in and out through your nose. Notice whether your chest feels or looks collapsed, or if it seems lifted. Don't try to change anything right away; just notice. Bring your fingers to rest on the two strong "cables" on either side of your neck, just beneath where your jawbones meet your ears. These cables are called the sternocleidomastoid muscles. They help to flex (draw forward) and rotate (turn) your head. You can feel these cables with your fingers, high up under your jaw, to see whether they are tight. If they are, you can hold or massage them as you breathe. For a couple of minutes, direct your breath to these cables. Use your breath to lengthen the area under your fingers. When you've released tension there, let go slowly.

Now, as you breathe, bring the pads (not tips) of your middle and ring fingers to the lymph node area right at the front of your throat and forward of the cables. Relax your fingers and bend them slightly, so you're not pressing into the side of your throat. Again, direct your breath to where your fingers are. Use your awareness and your breath to begin to generate space there. This may sound complex, but by simply breathing and relaxing you create less tension and more space.

When you feel sufficiently relaxed at the front of your throat, allow your throat to lengthen upward toward the ceiling. Provide the gentlest of guidance with your fingers. Keep "growing" your neck as long and tall as you can, like a giraffe's. Again, your finger pads should apply only the gentlest of pressure, so keep your fingers relaxed. Neck tension will interfere with this adjustment, so keep your neck loose as well. When you've reached maximum height, you'll find that your collarbones lift upward. Notice how much easier it is to breathe. Now you've gone "up the stairs."

Keep your shoulders steady (either against the wall, if you are at a wall, or in space, or in the mirror, if you're using one). Then, begin to draw your throat about one-quarter to one-half inch back behind you. Your shoulders may want to do the movement for you, so resist the urge to let them. Instead, focus on letting the movement come from your throat. If you are resting against a wall, you'll feel the back of your head come to touch the wall. If you're working with a mirror, you'll see the back of your head draw directly over your shoulders and upper spine. For the most part, this is not a large movement; only about half an inch, at most. Just remember to go upward (as you would go up a staircase backward) before going back. This is important, because your neck and throat can tighten if you go straight back without going upward first.

When you reach maximum movement back (or retraction), hold the finger pads gently on the lymph area at the front of the throat, and continue to breathe. Notice how much easier it is to breathe, to take in oxygen, now. Breathe in this position for several minutes. If you wish, you can relax your hands on your thighs or at your sides.

Feel the Difference

With your eyes closed, bring your attention to your body. Does it feel more energized, yet not overly so? Or does your body have excess energy? Are you somewhere in the middle? How does your mind feel? More alert, yet calm? Somewhere in between? Note any other responses. Do you feel lighter, for example? Do your emotions feel calmer? And which emotions come up in response to this pose? Record your observations in your notes. If at first you're not sure whether you're doing the pose correctly, or if you don't feel any different, stay with this exercise. Remember that your body is most likely integrating this adjustment, even if you can't feel it doing so. It can take ten times, or even more, for you to feel its impact.

4

Five Ways to Transform Your Emotional Patterns

In the mid-1980s, I began a doctoral program in biopsychology at the University of Chicago. My primary interest was the relationship between the mind and body. At about the same time, a pioneer psychologist at Harvard University was risking his reputation to explore the benefits of meditation on the mind and brain. Decades later, we crossed paths. By this point, Daniel Goleman's reputation was not only intact, it had flourished. Now a world-renowned author, he'd just published his latest book, *Social Intelligence*. Its topic was emotional contagion, our wired-in tendency to catch other people's positive and negative emotions. This interested me deeply, because I'd seen firsthand how Restorative Yoga helped people with one aspect of emotional balance: the ability to weather the emotional storms of loved ones without getting blown off course.

When we spoke, with great anticipation, I asked Daniel to name his top-three practices for emotional immunity. He immediately mentioned meditation, and cited many promising MRI studies on brain changes in long-term meditators. The passion in his voice stemmed both from the research and from his own long-standing meditation practice. But yoga, to my surprise, didn't even make his list. When I asked Daniel's opinion on yoga for emotional well-being, his answer caught me off guard: "Yoga is really just a form of physical exercise," he said. "Yoga in the *East*—now that's a different story." Daniel was referring to classical yoga, which is centered on the practice of meditation. Its principle text, and one of yoga's most widely read and respected works, is the Yoga Sutras, which mention the physical postures of yoga only three times. "The physical practice of yoga," Daniel said, "has one purpose: to get the body ready to sit in meditation." I asked what he thought about Restorative Yoga as a meditative practice. Yet at that point, Restorative Yoga had garnered very little attention here in the West compared with physically challenging forms of yoga. So, like many others in both the meditation and yoga communities, Dan hadn't yet heard of it. I described Restorative Yoga and talked about its ability to quiet the mind, balance the nervous system, *and* relax the body. "This sounds amazing," he said. "Why don't more people know about it?" Dan's question would ring in my ears for many months. Why *didn't* more people know about Restorative Yoga?

Since that conversation, I've heard many others in the Buddhist and meditation traditions express similar reservations about yoga. They feel that yoga bears little resemblance to a meditative practice. And in part, yoga deserves its poor stature in these communities. Here in the West, its reputation as a physical practice far eclipses its standing as a mental or contemplative one. Yoga has become a strength- and flexibility-building activity similar to exercise, and approximately sixteen million Americans practice it.[1]

Certainly, we can celebrate the physical practice of yoga on its own merit. It has a positive influence on nearly all the major systems of the body, including cardiovascular, circulatory, nervous, lymphatic, immune, muscular, skeletal, and endocrine. But yoga as a physical practice also increases brain levels of GABA (gamma-aminobutyric acid), an inhibitory neurotransmitter involved in anxiety and depression.[2] This is partly why it relieves stress and makes us feel less anxious and less depressed. The physical practice of yoga is also just enjoyable. It just feels good to move, to connect with our body, to become more conscious of our breath.

Although we can practice "physical yoga" and see emotional benefits, we can also use yoga's therapeutic elements mindfully to create emotional well-being. We can infuse the physical practice with therapeutic elements (such as slow transitions, mindful attention to alignment, and deeper breath). We can also supplement the physical practice with more meditative ones (regulated breathing, restorative postures, focused awareness of direct experience, and meditation). To do so successfully, however, we may need to adjust our tendency to overlook these subtle, meditative, and therapeutic aspects of yoga in favor of the more physical ones. From the time I first started teaching Restorative Yoga, I encouraged my students to embrace it as a stand-alone practice. Most, however, would only do it under one of two conditions: after a vigorous active practice (in which case they'd done their "workout" and could rationalize that they deserved it) or in response to an injury, illness, or stressful period (when they needed help or couldn't do an active practice).

Yet no matter the catalyst, I've seen remarkable things happen to people when they try Restorative Yoga. Those who did so after an active Vinyasa class experienced increased flexibility and energy. One man reported that his hips were more flexible than they were after attempting for years to open them through his active yoga practice. Those who tried it after an injury healed more quickly. A college student even repaired a foot fracture that her doctors said would need surgery. Those who tried Restorative Yoga for anxiety and depression felt emotionally stronger and more resilient. And several people told me that practicing late in the evening caused their sleeping to improve significantly. Some people have even brought restorative postures into their psychotherapy sessions and reported more transformative insight and change. One woman said that bringing restorative postures into her therapy helped her become aware of the endless stream of mental chatter and stories with which she'd hid her deeper issues. Once my students experienced Restorative Yoga's remarkable effects on the mind, body, and emotions, most made it a regular part of their practice.

There's a reason why I didn't choose active yoga postures for this book. The yoga tools featured here combine mental and contemplative practices with body-based ones. These tools (breathing exercises, focused awareness, and Restorative Yoga) have a stronger therapeutic influence on emotional healing than either mental or physical practices alone. They also impact the body directly, while most traditional meditative practices do so more indirectly. These tools become especially powerful because the nervous system is in the body. The breath is in the body. The present moment is in the body. The mind is in the body. We even filter emotional experience through the body. Combining yoga's meditative practices with the native wisdom of the body makes our mental and physical work more integrative, and amplifies its benefits.

Someday, the practice of yoga in the West will emphasize yoga's meditative elements as strongly as its physical ones. The mindfulness and meditation communities may then perceive more common ground with yoga. These fields could even collaborate to bring more evolution to the mind *and* body together. Until then, yoga therapy can point the way toward an exploration of yoga as a valid form of *body-based meditation*.

We've examined the roots of emotional imbalance in the mind, body, and nervous system. We've looked at how practicing old behaviors prevents change. We've also explored how the careful sequencing of therapeutic tools helps emotional healing happen in a more progressive, integrated way. Now we're ready to take an intimate look at the five building blocks for lasting healing:

1. Balancing the nervous system
2. Regulating the breath
3. Cultivating direct experience
4. Quieting the mind
5. Changing our personal narratives

Notice that none of these elements involves a vigorous physical yoga practice—not even a Downward Dog pose. Each of these elements draws from the more meditative and therapeutic aspects of yoga. If you're used to a purely physical practice, or on the other hand to not doing much with your body at all, this may necessitate a shift in the way you approach yoga and emotional health. Yet once you embrace these subtle healing practices and witness how well they create change, you'll be able to re-create this change in other areas of your life.

These five elements build beautifully in a progressive sequence; each one becomes a foundation for the next. These elements help reduce our emotional reactivity. They restabilize us after strong emotional reactions. They build on one another well. They lend themselves well to repetition (or neuroplasticity) and thus to permanent positive changes in the mind and body. And once we've begun to internalize them, we can use them in any active yoga practice, psychotherapy session, or life situation to become more centered and emotionally healthy.

1. Balancing the Nervous System

The nervous system excels at neuroplasticity, at building experience. It acts as a foundation for the development of the other four therapeutic elements of yoga. The nervous system is an emotional intermediary; it filters all of our emotional experiences. Nervous system balance requires a kind of emotional elasticity: the ability to react when necessary, but not overreact, and the ability to return fluidly to a healthy emotional baseline. So nervous system balance, then, is a prerequisite for emotional balance.

Your Own Inner Calming System

As I've described, your nervous system responds in much the same way to strong emotions as it does to acute stress: by going into overdrive. In anxiety and depression, the fight-flight-freeze branch of the nervous system speeds up with very little prompting. Normally, the relaxation branch of the nervous system puts the brakes on this response. But in both anxiety and depression, it doesn't slow things down quickly or efficiently enough. This creates a chronic fight-flight-freeze or stress response.

Imagine that your emergency response system turns on all the lights in your house (your nervous system). From half a block away, you can see the lights blazing. While you wouldn't want to waste energy by constantly leaving all the lights on all the time, you wouldn't want to turn them all completely off, either. To interact with others and respond to daily life, you need to be a little reactive; you need some lights on. But are you activated and anxious or depressed most of the time? To conserve energy and preserve your health, you need a "dimmer switch." Then *you* can control the lighting.

Luckily, your brain has a built-in dimmer switch: the parasympathetic (rest-and-digest) system. While the sympathetic nervous system gets you agitated, the parasympathetic system calms you. It lowers heart rate, blood pressure, respiration rate, and stress hormones. It increases digestion and strengthens immune function. In contrast to the fight-flight-freeze response, the rest-and-digest system conserves rather than expends your energy, and revitalizes rather than depletes you. When the lights (your sympathetic system's arousal levels) are too intense, your parasympathetic branch dims them and calms you down. It acts as "mood lighting."

While it might sound as though these two systems work against each other, that's not the case; the sympathetic and parasympathetic systems actually function in synergy. When the sympathetic is in charge, you react quickly to things and feel more anxious or depressed. When the parasympathetic system dominates, you overreact less and feel more calm and emotionally grounded. When these two systems are working together, they're like partners: they create a state of dynamic equilibrium and exchange.

At a workshop not long ago, a young man raised his hand to announce that he didn't have a parasympathetic nervous system. Although his fellow participants responded with good-natured laughter, he had a point: sometimes it can feel as though, like missing an arm or a leg, you were born without a rest-and-digest system, without the capacity to relax. But no matter how long you've felt anxious or depressed, you were born with your rest-and-digest system, or dimmer switch, intact. This means that *you have an innate capacity for relaxation*, which is the foundation of emotional balance. You just may not have used your dimmer switch—your parasympathetic system's relaxation response—enough to wire its pattern in more strongly than your habitual anxiety or depression one.

To become more emotionally balanced, you first need to learn how to access your parasympathetic system in nonstressful situations. This is important; it strengthens neural pathways to relaxation and calm when you're not emotionally stirred up. With repetition, these new pathways become stronger, more mature. Then they're able to compete with the less healthy, more reactive ones. With practice, you learn the trick of accessing and using your dimmer switch when you experience an emotional reaction. Then you become like Hansel and Gretel: you can leave a trail of "emotional bread crumbs" to help you use these pathways in emotionally charged situations such as a knock-down, drag-out family fight or a difficult breakup. This will help you find your way out of the woods and back to emotional balance in nearly any intense situation. Eventually you'll become proficient at it: you'll be able to increase arousal levels (when you want more response) and decrease them (when you need more calm).

You might be wondering how to do this. How do you engage your emotional dimmer switch? The key is relaxation, an inherent part of breathing exercises and Restorative Yoga.

Relaxation

For many people, the term *relaxation* connotes "chilling out," taking time to do nothing. The command "Relax!" is now a trendy way to tell someone to give you a break or to "chill out." But chilling out doesn't necessarily mean that you're relaxed. While you're watching TV, for example, your body can be at ease while your mind and nervous system remain highly engaged. This combination—relaxed body, amped-up mind—echoes mixed anxiety and depression. It actually discourages relaxation and healing.

True relaxation is deeply therapeutic, and involves muscular relaxation in the body *and* quieting, or lowered emotional reactivity, in the mind. Your brain waves, a measure of your brain's activity level, are slower during relaxation than during active wakefulness, yet more active than in sleep. This state helps you focus your awareness on an element of the breath, a part of the body, or a pattern of thought or emotion. Restorative Yoga is an ideal way to create true relaxation.

Restorative Yoga

Here's how Restorative Yoga works: While muscular tension activates the sympathetic nervous system, Restorative Yoga uses props in each pose to minimize muscle tension and maximize physical comfort and relaxation. While sensory stimulation (light, sound, touch, and so forth) activates the fight-flight-freeze response, Restorative Yoga is done in a reasonably warm, dimly lit, and quiet room to reduce sensory stimulation and keep the nervous system calm. While sitting and standing postures elevate heart rate and blood pressure (which can heighten nervous system arousal), Restorative Yoga postures keep the head at or below the level of the heart to reduce heart rate and blood pressure and quiet the nervous system. While a longer inhalation and breathing through the mouth can trigger hyperventilation (which increases heart rate and mental activity), Restorative Yoga incorporates nasal breathing (and in particular, a longer exhalation) to lower heart rate and nervous system activity.

Years ago, I participated in a television series on alternative health. The show focused on Restorative Yoga for insomnia. The producer asked me an interesting question, one I've heard many times since: "What's the difference between Restorative Yoga and sleep? Why can't you just take a nap with a pillow under your head to balance your emotions?" If it were this easy, I sometimes tell people, we'd all be emotionally balanced.

Restorative Yoga is different from sleep. Psychologist and sleep researcher Roger Cole also teaches yoga in California. As he points out, during ordinary (non–rapid eye movement) sleep, brain waves slow to unconsciousness while the body relaxes. Yet the body's relaxation can be less profound when you're asleep than when you're in a state of true relaxation.[3] A friend of mine recently confided that she'd awakened one morning to find herself rigid in a backbend, the crown of her head actively pressing into her pillow; another friend grinds his teeth at night. You can take your stress to bed with you, which means that your muscles stay tense, even in sleep, and your stress hormones elevate. So sleep may not be as relaxing as we think it is.

Restorative Yoga allows your nervous system to balance and your body to relax while your brain remains in a state of alert observation. This state is helpful; it allows you to react less intensely to your thoughts and emotions and to regain your balance more quickly after they pass. Because Restorative Yoga involves the body as well as the mind, its meditative and relaxing benefits can be embodied rather than just mentally understood. As an example, Suzanne, a yoga therapy client, utilized Restorative Yoga to move out of her constant "fight mode" and into a calmer place in her relationship with her mind and body, and with her boyfriend.

Suzanne frequently found herself enraged at her boyfriend. Something he'd do, which she'd later admit was minor, always prompted it. Coming home a little later than he promised, going out with the guys, or talking with his mouth full inspired in Suzanne a full-blown case of what a friend calls "Sudden Repulsion Syndrome." Without warning, she'd become sickened by everything he did, and she'd lash out in rage. Inevitably, her anger would shadow her to work, the gym, and home again. Each time her nervous system would begin to relax, she'd kick it back into high gear, inventing arguments with him in her head until she was trembling with fury. While this took its toll on both of them, Suzanne paid the higher price. Her boyfriend usually let go of the conflict within a couple of hours; it left his mind and body. But Suzanne couldn't put the brakes on. She would spend the next two days marinating in anger. These episodes produced stomach pain significant enough on occasion to bring her to the emergency room.

Although Suzanne recognized that her constant anger and anxiety were making her sick and ruining her relationship with her boyfriend, this insight hadn't changed a thing. But in yoga therapy, Suzanne learned to bring awareness to the sequence of events in her anxiety cycle, starting with the trigger (her boyfriend acting in a way she couldn't control). She noted the hyperactive and worried thoughts that indicate mental anxiety: *Why does he have to do that? I've asked him not to a thousand times. He'll probably leave the house without saying good-bye, which he knows I hate. . . .* She also observed the strong sense of internal pressure (a racing heart, fidgeting, pacing back and forth, and shortness of breath) that signaled agitation in her body. She didn't try to "think" her way out of this pattern by using positive thoughts. Instead, she added therapeutic yoga techniques to interrupt this cycle as early as possible. She addressed the agitation in her mind and nervous system through breathing: When her thoughts would begin to accelerate, she'd practice 1:2 Breathing (page 72) to calm her mind. Then she'd choose a pose from the anxiety-balancing sequence (see chapter 8) to relax and slow down her body. With practice, Suzanne experienced only a mild irritation with her boyfriend and was able to manage it better.

2. Regulating the Breath

The second way to balance our emotions is to breathe fully and deeply. When we regulate our breathing and make it slower and deeper, the rest-and-digest system becomes more dominant. Conversely, when we don't regulate our breathing, and breathe shallowly, the nervous system moves into hyperarousal mode—just what we don't want.

Conscious breathing is essential to emotional balance. Rapid and shallow breathing, which most people do, hinders the body's response to emotion and stress. It slows the circulation of oxygen in the brain, muscles, and tissue. It constricts blood vessels and reduces blood to the brain and muscles; over time, this can lead to heart disease, stroke, and other illnesses. Rapid, shallow breathers usually breathe through their mouths; this stimulates hyperventilation and activates the nervous system. Even when someone feels emotionally balanced, rapid and shallow breathing can trigger a bout of anxiety and stress. Rapid and shallow breathing contributes to the elevated nervous system arousal we see in both anxiety and depression.

In contrast, slow and deep breathing improves the body's response to emotional stress. It increases the circulation of oxygen in the brain, muscles, and tissue. Slow, deep breathing dilates blood vessels and improves digestion. Slow and deep breathers breathe through their nose; this helps deepen the breath and reduce hyperventilation which, in turn, helps the nervous system to relax. Even when someone feels emotionally off center, just breathing slowly and deeply can stimulate the relaxation response, reducing anxiety and stress. Slow, deep, regulated breathing balances the nervous system and quiets the mind, which helps develop healthier emotional patterns.

William, one of my students, found breathing to be a big challenge. He'd spent most of his adult life battling depression and anxiety. Each morning he'd awaken to find himself covered by a blanket of lethargy so intense that he could barely get out of bed. His mind, however, constantly worried. Like many people, William breathed in and out through his mouth, quite shallowly. It took two months of twice-weekly sessions to train William to breathe through his nose. When he got the hang of it, he experienced a dramatic increase in mental calm, and yet the restorative poses energized his body. He felt a sense of hope and possibility that he hadn't felt in twenty-five years.

One of the best and easiest ways to regulate your breathing is to breathe in *and* out through your nose. Nasal breathing is deeper than mouth breathing. In nasal breathing, the exhale is naturally longer than the inhale. This lowers heart rate, which in turn *calms the nervous system.* Surprising as it may sound, deep nasal breathing helps you worry less. If nasal breathing alone, which makes the exhale slightly longer, helps the mind and nervous system so much, imagine what happens when you make the exhale considerably longer, which you do during 1:2 Breathing.

In a recent teacher-training session, I had my students experiment directly with the breath's influence on the mind and nervous system. I instructed them to choose a partner and discuss something stressful for five minutes. Soon, they began to fidget. Their eyes grew more activated, approximating the "Olive Oyl" alertness of anxiety. Each student rated his or her level of anxiety, which rose dramatically during the five-minute discussions. I then guided them through several rounds of 1:2 Breathing, with the exhale twice as long as the inhale. After several minutes, everyone reported a dramatic drop in anxiety. This made sense, but I wanted to know more. If slow, deep breathing could reverse an episode of anxiety already in progress, would those calming benefits continue if anxiety were reintroduced?

To explore this further, I had my students return to their 1:2 breathing pattern and revisit their stressful thoughts. Most reported that although their breathing remained steady and they exhaled twice as long as they inhaled, something strange happened: they simply couldn't muster up the same level of anxiety they'd had before. The few who said they had gotten worried suddenly realized that they'd lost the 1:2 breathing ratio. In other words, 1:2 breathing creates a mental state largely incompatible with anxiety. The next time you feel deeply anxious or stressed out, try 1:2 Breathing, or let your exhale be longer than your inhale. You'll find yourself calmer within minutes.

Breathwork, the practice of regulating your breath, is a powerful tool. It isn't just one of those things you'd do in a formal yoga practice or on those rare occasions when you have some extra time on your hands. Like Restorative Yoga, breathwork is *immediately and directly helpful* in lowering your emotional reactivity. B. K. S. Iyengar, who founded the Iyengar style of yoga, practiced several hours of breathwork daily, well into his nineties, because he experienced its benefits firsthand and witnessed them in his students. You can practice breathing exercises at work to help manage your stress. You can use breathwork at home to help you be a less emotionally reactive parent or partner. Or try 1:2 Breathing (see page 72) if you have insomnia and want to fall asleep more quickly. You can even do breathwork in the middle of a fight, when it can calm you down and help you generate more empathy for a potential "emotional enemy." Focusing on the breath also has a fringe benefit: it helps you reside in the present moment, and not the past or future.

3. Cultivating Direct Experience

The third way to change emotional patterns is to cultivate direct experience of the present moment and of your body. You might be wondering what *not* being in the moment (or in your body) could possibly have to do with anxiety and depression. Or how being *in* the moment (or in the body) can contribute to emotional balance. As a client once commented testily, "I don't have the time or luxury to get all 'Zen' about my depression." But because of its close relationship to anxiety and depression, present-moment awareness isn't, as my client implied, a New Age concept. Emotional balance has a lot to do with how centered we are in the body and how closely we pay attention to what's happening right now, in the moment.

Becoming Present in the Body

Both types of awareness, body awareness and present-moment awareness, are intimately connected. The body is our best teacher on the subject of present-moment awareness. It doesn't worry about the future or fixate on the past. It doesn't concern itself with how it looks or question whether it is loved. The body just *is*. When we're out of our body, we're also often "out of time," or not in the present moment—since being in the body and being connected to the present go hand in hand.

Think for a moment how easy it is to go through an entire day not really feeling your body or being aware of it. Usually, when you're not *in* your body, you're in your head or mind instead. But here's the thing: anxiety and depression have roots in the body. So when you don't inhabit the body, it's hard to change these patterns.

For Cameron, one of my students, yoga was a revelation. A music professor in his midsixties, Cameron had difficulty being in his body. He was extremely intelligent, and lived much more in his mind. As a result, Cameron had trouble identifying physical sensations such as fatigue, pain, or relaxation. He often mixed up the right and left sides of his body, or had trouble moving an arm or a leg as instructed in yoga class. Sometimes, Cameron had minor accidents while writing symphonies in his head, and crashed into furniture or broke things. He gamely endured his physical awkwardness and occasional falls in class. Within a year, he began to see rewards from his persistence. He started to experience his body in a different way: not as something that was aging or betraying him, but as an instrument of ease and grace. Every month or so, during an active practice, his eyes would open wide and he'd look at me with a huge grin, astonished to see himself doing something new. As hard as it was for him to grow older, his blossoming friendship with his body seemed to ease the process of aging. Cameron stayed

centered in his body more often, whether he was having a graceful experience or a clumsy one, a contented day or a difficult one.
This direct presence in his body also helped his mental outlook. He
softened his tendency to beat himself up for nearly everything. His
bouts of melancholy and artist's block grew much less frequent.
Cameron learned that just connecting to direct experience—even
in a not-so-very-young, not-so-very-graceful, not-so-very-comfort-
able body—built a foundation for emotional health.

Nervous system imbalance and stress create tension and pain in
the body, which makes the body more likely to hold on to difficult
emotional patterns. The chronic nervous system imbalance and
stress we experience in anxiety and depression can make the body
feel like a battleground. Naturally, we don't want to inhabit the
battleground of the anxious or depressed body fully. This starts out
as a protective mechanism: the body feels pain, discomfort. Focusing on direct experience can temporarily amplify this discomfort.
So to escape, we try to "leave" the body, to dissociate. We draw
our awareness right out of the body and focus it elsewhere. When
people have a serious accident or endure tremendous physical pain,
you might hear them say afterward that they floated outside their
body or went "somewhere else."

In anxiety and depression, dissociation is a common strategy designed to protect us from difficult feelings. Yet this strategy doesn't
work so well. It ceases to be a self-protective, short-term emergency
reaction and can become a self-abandoning, long-term one. Disso-
ciating from the body has major consequences. Not being in the
body prevents us from actually feeling, which is the first step in developing emotional balance. And not being in the body means that
we miss the feeling of victory, the sense of strength and belief in
ourselves that come from being present with and working through
painful emotions. What's more, not being in the body keeps us from
having and repeating new, positive experiences. So if we're not in
the body when we practice yoga, we won't integrate the energy and
expansiveness we'd find in a depression-lifting practice, or the calm
and grounding we'd encounter in an anxiety-balancing one. What
happens then? These new sensations leak away, replaced by the
very discomfort we hoped to avoid. Even though it starts out as

a protective mechanism, dissociation usually makes things worse by alienating us from ourselves. At the same time, suffering from anxiety, depression, or trauma can cause people to get used to not being in their body. If this sounds like you, or you haven't been able to be present in your body for a long time, you may find it at first uncomfortable to reconnect. For this reason, the exercises in each chapter of part 1 of this book guide you through that process in a gradual, yet progressive way.

If we're not present in our body, we can't lay down the building blocks for emotional change. Radha, a student who endured painful war trauma and suffered from post-traumatic stress disorder, recently approached me after class to ask for a referral. Thinking she meant for psychotherapy, I began to tell her of the psychotherapists I know who work well with trauma. "Oh no," she told me. "Been there, done that. It helped. But I don't want to talk *about* my experiences anymore. I just want to work *with* my body." Since practicing yoga, she told me, she'd begun to feel a hint of peace, and wanted to continue her internal "cease-fire." She knew it would be painful, but she felt that the road to healing actually wound into and through her body.

Whether our pain is physical or mental, acute or chronic, we can learn to anchor ourselves in direct experience of the body. Doing so rewards us. From direct experience, we learn to listen to the body and hear what it needs. For example, the constant tension we feel in the company of people we care about may signal a need for time alone. The abdominal tension we have every time we enter our office may signal the need for a new job. The contagious effects of our fights with loved ones may tell us that we really desire less combative relationships, or more compassion. The body may even crave a few minutes of deep breathing or time spent relaxing in a restorative pose. Through our direct experience, we begin to pay attention, and we learn. What would happen if you inhabited and listened to your body? What do you think it would say to you?

The exercises in the first part of this book are a great opportunity to experience the instructive nature of direct body experience. As you do these exercises, you'll encounter sensations, both pleasant and unpleasant. Try to stay present with them. You can focus on the breath, which is neither positive nor negative. You can focus on a part of your body, which is also neither good nor bad. You can even use your breath to channel difficult emotional experiences through your body. You don't need to process or mentally understand what happens in the body or why. All your body requires of you is presence, and allowing. When you cultivate direct experience of your body no matter what's happening, you develop friendliness toward it. Then, when things get really tough, such as in situations of extreme emotional pain, your body becomes an ally.

Becoming Rooted in the Moment

Staying rooted in direct experience of the moment can be a challenge. We tend to treat time as an adversary; we can never get enough of it. We race against it, and try to bend it to our will. And the way we relate to time affects our emotional well-being. In an anxiety pattern, awareness typically hooks on to the future and not the here and now. We're likely to spend considerable energy worrying about things that haven't happened yet: *If I don't come home on time, is she going to freak out again? What if I can't fall asleep tonight? Where should I go for lunch today—and do I have time to get there and back?* We may also interpret ordinary events as signs of impending danger. When we dwell on the future in a negative way, we "rehearse" anxiety. We create more of it.

In depression, awareness gets stuck in the quicksand of the past more often than it stays centered in the present. We tend to revisit and replay, over and over, painful things that have already happened. *Why did he leave me? What's wrong with me? Why did I have to say such a stupid thing? I'm sure I just drove him away.* We may filter our experiences with negativity and pessimism. The tendency to obsess about the past and focus on the negative repeats our depression pattern. It also brings more negativity, more suffering, into the future.

How can yoga help? Sure, it's possible to practice yoga and still fixate on the future or obsess about the past. Yet *being present* is a central focus of yoga. Yoga invites us to be present in several ways. It brings us right into our mind and emotions, just as they are this very moment. It links us with our breath, just as it is now.

It connects us with our body, no matter what shape or form it takes at present.

Not long ago Willa, a regular Restorative Yoga student, approached me at the beginning of class to say she wasn't sure if she should be there at all. Breathlessly, she told me that she'd just had a breast biopsy earlier that day. She was filled with apprehension. Should she just come back, Willa wondered, after she got the results? I encouraged her to stay, and alerted my assistants to have a box of Kleenex on hand in case she needed them. But after ten minutes of restless settling in, she "dropped in" to her body and appeared to be at peace. Willa moved very little, staying in one pose for most of her practice. After class she came up, flushed with excitement. "I never realized before," she said, "how quickly Restorative Yoga helps me let go of what's going on in the outside world!" Willa practiced restorative poses every day throughout her ordeal, which included another minor procedure. She did this not to forget what was happening in her life, but to stay centered. She wanted to build a sense of inner calm that would remain steady, no matter what the rest of her life held.

Yoga gives you a task—focusing—that's all-consuming. So all-consuming that it can interrupt, as it did for Willa, your preoccupation with the past or future. When you root yourself in the moment, and in your body, something else happens: you uproot your focus from anxiety and depression. You have an *embodied* experience of . . . being *not* anxious or *not* depressed! The body and mind remember this sensation; each time it occurs, you strengthen the healthier (not anxious and not depressed) pattern.

When I first began to do yoga therapy, I wondered if this direct experience of the moment and the body would be accessible to everyone. Could people with chronic anxiety and depression practice it and benefit? Could older people, who tend to dwell more in the past? I watched my father, who began yoga at the age of eighty, to see how the "direct experience" part of the practice impacted him. For my dad, the phrase *being in the moment* wouldn't have entered a conversation. He thought it was New Age jargon, and definitely not the kind of thing that could help him. After he started yoga, though, I noted how his relationship with time changed. Dad became happier, even more engaged with life than before. He found enjoyment in the moment: monitoring the daily arguments and flight patterns of sparrows outside his window, supervising the browning of his sourdough bread in the toaster oven, watching clouds trek across the sky, or scanning, with a magnifying glass, baby pictures of his daughter and his grandson for similarities. The more connected to the moment he was, the more upbeat and positive he became. Being in the moment also helped Dad to be more present in his body. He could describe physical sensations more clearly, and access parts of his body through yoga that he couldn't before, such as his hamstrings. More importantly, connecting with his direct experience helped Dad navigate his physical challenges with grace.

Dad's ability to be in the present taught me about myself. Often, I'd budget a certain amount of time for his yoga sessions or for spending time together. I'd try to fit these visits into a part of my day, rushing to get to him and rushing out to get to someplace else. But there was no way to hurry him: a yoga class or a visit sitting outside together, sharing the *New York Times* and eating ice cream, took as long it took. Dad so immersed himself in his present moment experience that he lost track of time. Some days, this made me anxious. I'd think: *How will I get my work done on time? How far behind will this put me?* Almost every visit, I overextended my "allotted time" with him. Yet each time, I'd return to work to find myself more at peace, more able to accomplish what I needed. This gave me unexpected emotional benefits: for one thing, a greater sense of well-being. For another, a more relaxed and deeper connection to myself. Spending time with older people, young children, or in nature has this same effect: it yokes us to the present, which is really where it's at.

Balancing the nervous system, deepening the breath, and cultivating awareness of our direct body-centered and present-moment experience all build emotional balance. Surprisingly, they can also help quiet the mind. How does this work, and what's the mechanism by which it happens?

4. Quieting the Mind

The fourth way to change emotional patterns is to quiet the mind. In breathing and restorative practices, we don't have the "blessing" of movement to distract the mind like we do in an active physical practice. I've experienced the challenge of this stillness myself. Years ago, when sensory deprivation tanks were popular, I signed up for a few sessions. I'd change into a bathing suit, put on my goggles, and climb into the slightly-larger-than-coffin-sized saltwater tank. At first the warm water, complete lack of sound, and utter darkness would feel comforting, even luxurious. Not too long into the session, though, my mind would find the utter quiet unsettling. Without the distractions of light and sound, thoughts weren't enough. I'd begin to have the most vivid, lifelike hallucinations. At the time, it unnerved me a little. Later, I learned that because the mind has such a hard time doing nothing, hallucinations are a common side effect of sensory deprivation.

In Restorative Yoga, the body is still. We reduce sensory stimulation (such as light, sound, even touch). For the mind, this is when the hard part can begin. Just as the mind doesn't trust the body to do things "right" in our daily lives, it may not trust the body in Restorative Yoga, either. It can keep up an incessant barrage of concerns: *What's going on? Why isn't something happening? I don't feel any better. This stuff is not working.* Without something to anchor to, the mind becomes incredibly inventive and can conjure things out of thin air. The yoga tradition affectionately calls this tendency "monkey mind."

No matter what the body is doing, the mind is agile and can jump from one branch of thought to the next. My student Mia found this out when she discovered meditation halfway through her second year of practicing yoga. She threw herself into it wholeheartedly, signing up for a two-week silent yoga and meditation retreat just before Labor Day. The first day of the retreat, after a vigorous physical practice, she sat quietly. For six hours, as she tried to focus her mind, she mentally redecorated her house. She felt happy, excited to see the wonderful things she'd done to beautify her living space. In the back of her mind, though, she felt slightly guilty for not quieting her mind more. On the second day, Mia's mind occupied the first three hours by cataloguing her boyfriend's flaws, and then moved on to all the things that were wrong in their relationship. With clarity, she realized that she had to break up with him as soon as the retreat was over. She felt sad and hopeless. Would she ever find someone to love, who loved her back the way she deserved? The third day, Mia's mind returned to her newly decorated home and made a few changes: *How could I have chosen salmon for the living room?* she wondered. In the afternoon, her thoughts returned to her relationship. She was surprised to discover a sense of understanding, even tenderness, toward her boyfriend. Why hadn't she realized before how caring and loyal he was? She felt happy and resolved to appreciate him more. *We should get married,* she decided, and the wedding planning lasted into the night and partway through the next morning's meditation. Over the remainder of the retreat, Mia's mind followed its busy schedule. In the midst of one of several imaginary breakups with her boyfriend, she even fell deeply in love with the long-haired guy on the meditation cushion in front of her (she couldn't see his face, but he just "radiated attractiveness!"). When she returned home after her ten-day retreat, having finally achieved some measure of mental quiet, she'd been married three times (to two different men), divorced twice, and had redecorated no less than five times. Mia marveled at the tenacity of the human mind, at its inventiveness in creating such vivid mental and emotional experiences. She learned firsthand how the mind fluctuates constantly, especially when the body is still. But she also learned to observe these fluctuations as both a natural occurrence and as a prelude to quiet. Yoga philosophy discusses the fluctuations of the mind at great length, even stating that stilling these fluctuations is the definitive goal of yoga.[4]

The meditative and therapeutic elements of yoga can help with these fluctuations. In Restorative Yoga, the body remains fairly still, except when changing postures. At first, our mind may pick up speed, grasping at everything it can. Yet when we focus on direct experience, we see how experience changes from moment to moment. The mind witnesses these fluctuations in direct experience. It watches physical pain come and go. It sees sadness arrive and depart. It feels pride wax and wane. It senses worry course through us and then pass. Then it settles down and quiets. The next time we practice, we go through the same cycle: the mind accelerates and then quiets. We begin to sense the rhythm of the mind. We see its fluctuations as a natural tendency, and they become less alluring, less convincing. The quiet starts to gain ground; we begin to integrate it, to access it even in the midst of troubling situations. When we do, we change the way we filter and react to these situations. Even our personal narratives begin to change.

5. Changing Our Personal Narratives

The fifth way to change emotional patterns is to observe, and eventually shift, the way we filter our direct experience. This filter can reveal itself clearly in the narratives we tell ourselves and others. Changing these narratives may be difficult; sometimes, they act as a mechanism for social bonding. Have you ever stood in a long line at the post office, say, on April fifteenth, with someone whose loud sighs and muttered comments invited you to join in complaint about the long wait or the evils of government? Or gotten into a "whose circumstances are more challenging" contest with a friend to see who deserves the most sympathy? We tell stories to connect with others. We use them to give and receive support. We share them to let people know that we suffer, too. We may hope that, in exchange, they won't be intimidated by us.

Though they emphasize storytelling, psychotherapy, support groups, and retreat centers offer tremendous value. Part of their value lies in catharsis: the release that comes when we voice our past and share our feelings about it. When we reveal something we've been unable to express, we feel empowered. The process of revelation—of being heard, seen, and validated by others—is deeply affirming. For the first several dozen times we tell it, our story has value. And then something happens to the story. It gets rehearsed. And rehearsed . . . and rehearsed . . . until it becomes a powerful samskara of its own.

When the story is a positive one, it helps the mind, body, and nervous system. Yet when it's negative, pessimistic, suspicious, or self-critical, it can engrave anxiety and depression more deeply into us. Recently Lisa, a yoga therapy client, came to me for fertility issues. She told me she'd gone to a support group once and never returned. The name of the group was the "Infertility Group," she said, which made her think about her "problem body." Not surprisingly, the stories shared by her fellow group members revolved around themes of damaged bodies and broken dreams. They focused on difficult medical and emotional experiences. These stories were in some ways accurate; nonetheless, they caused Lisa's mood to dip considerably. She left the first session so down that she had difficulty getting out of bed for two days afterward.

We can give our power away to our stories. We can let them become our personal myths. They can gain so much momentum that they become incredibly hard to change. And unfortunately, our stories have an unintended effect of spreading to the rest of the mind-body network. Once there, they cause a cascade of neurobiological (brain- and body-related) events that amplify nervous system activation and through it, anxiety and depression. This means that, as we learned in chapters 1 and 2, telling stories about our pain can actually cause us to practice pain, and to increase it.

To observe our stories with detachment is difficult; to release our stories, even more so. Yet in this as well, Restorative Yoga offers a solution. Restorative Yoga turns on your dimmer switch. It balances your nervous system. It quiets the mind. Through breathwork, focused awareness, and relaxation, it brings you deep into direct experience. These benefits help you see your stories from a new perspective. You observe them as mental and emotional fluctuations. Restorative Yoga makes you more reflective about your experiences, as I learned with Rachael, one of my early clients.

When Rachael first came to see me for yoga therapy, her well-entrenched bouts of anxiety and anger interfered with her work and personal life. These episodes came with a side order of insomnia and low self-esteem. Rachael already practiced yoga and felt that it helped her with her emotions. She wanted to manage her anxiety the "natural way" rather than take the Xanax her doctor had prescribed. Our weekly sessions began with a brief update on her life. Then we moved to active yoga (mainly Sun Salutations) and ended with an anxiety-balancing restorative practice. Rachael quickly learned the sequence of postures and practiced on her own. I expected Restorative Yoga to help with her nervous system balance, and it did: within weeks, her anxiety dissipated and she could sleep better. Perhaps most remarkable, however, was something I never anticipated. In the beginning of her sessions, while she was sitting upright and giving me an update on her life, Rachael's stories were flavored with judgment and blame. Her boyfriend Geoff was really a jerk in disguise "just like all the guys" she dated. Her "less intelligent" colleagues bugged her (no one was as special, as uniquely talented, as she was). Her sister Sara was jealous of her. I'd heard these kinds of stories from clients for years. For the most part, their telling and retelling didn't seem to relieve anxiety or depression.

Yet as soon as Rachael moved into the active, body-centered part of the session, something shifted. During Sun Salutations, she became focused on integrating her movement and breath. She seemed visibly calmer and less angry. The biggest change, however, came within minutes of moving into Restorative Yoga: Rachael's talking slowed down considerably. She stopped processing her interactions with others in a negative, cyclical way. She viewed the people in her life (the loser boyfriend, incompetent radiologist, ignorant co-workers, and annoying sister) with less reactivity and more compassion. Her thinking grew more conducive to finding creative solutions. Rachael astounded me when, twenty minutes into her third restorative session, she came up with a wise insight: by pressuring her boyfriend to stay in and not go out with friends, she was smothering him. In response, he naturally wanted to "burst out" of his confinement. "If I'd just give him a little space," she mused, "he'd probably be more demonstrative."

Initially, I suspected that this was a onetime transformation, an example of "instant healing" that would disappear as suddenly as it had come. Yet each time Rachael dropped into a restorative pose, these insightful moments recurred. They weren't just mental insights but embodied ones, and they began to change how Rachael viewed and related to her world. She started to soften toward others. She generated more empathy when Geoff or her friends didn't comply with her demands. Soon, she began to connect her harsh judgment of others with her lack of compassion toward herself: not in an "insight-in-the-mind" kind of way but in a more embodied, lasting way. Even then, I wondered whether this transformation might be unique to Rachael. I thought it could be a fortuitous blossoming of spirit or a happy therapeutic "accident." Since then, however, I've seen this with hundreds of clients.

Restorative Yoga and How You Think

Restorative Yoga benefits you on an *intra*personal (internal) level. It doesn't just help you rest and digest physically; it helps you do so emotionally as well. It makes it easier to digest your emotions, learn from them, and then let them go. In an active yoga practice, the body is so engaged that the mind has less space for reflection. In Restorative Yoga, the body is relaxed. The nervous system is quieter and the mind is more reflective, all *while you're feeling your emotions*. Because the body is relaxed, you can experience feelings of anger, sadness, or worry more fully and with less reactivity than you might in either a meditation or an active yoga practice. What's more, your body integrates these experiences. In these ways, the parasympathetic system is like a "reflect-and-redirect" system. It helps you reflect on your experiences. It redirects your thoughts and emotions. It promotes embodied insight.

Restorative Yoga benefits you interpersonally, as well. The restorative practice has an amazing effect on the way you think. How does it do this? It turns on your dimmer switch and calms your nervous system. This allows you to observe your intense emotional reactions and negative thought patterns *while you're in a state of deep relaxation.* Because you're relaxed, it's hard for you to get worried or caught up in what's bothering you. How can you? Your nervous system and body are at ease. So you begin to look at emotionally charged issues with greater perspective. You come to understand better why people do the things they do (as Rachael did with her boyfriend). Instead of beating yourself up, you may gain more self-compassion. You may become more mindful and reflective. You may see your old stories as less interesting, even less compelling. You start to see the ways in which they are inaccurate or self-limiting. Sooner or later, you stop telling them as often. When your old stories lose their pull, new stories—new ways of processing interactions and experiences—can emerge.

Recently, a teacher-training student asked whether the benefits of Restorative Yoga (increased understanding, compassion, capacity for reflection, and nonjudgment) translate into our everyday interactions. The answer is yes. The embodied insight in Restorative Yoga doesn't need a teacher or yoga therapist to keep it going. It grows and develops in its own rhythm, practice after practice. This embodied insight lasts longer than mental insight and also spreads into your life beyond the practice.

Restorative Yoga helps you develop many of the characteristics of emotional balance, such as the ability to experience emotions without overreacting to them, and the capacity to recover from strong emotions when they occur. It supports the qualities that psychotherapy seeks to instill: greater resourcefulness, enhanced problem-solving skills, and a deeper connection with your innate wisdom. It helps you develop the mindfulness, discernment, and reflection that lead to healthier relationships.

Sometimes it can feel as if the struggle for emotional balance is an uphill one. We can compare ourselves to people who seem more evolved than we are. On top of this, we are besieged by glossy magazine images of seemingly effortless equanimity and calm. We may feel like Sisyphus, the mythical king punished with the task of rolling a boulder uphill, only to have it roll down again and repeat the process throughout eternity. We may fear that like Sisyphus, we'll always be dragging the burden of our emotions up a giant mountain, only to have them lose control and make us begin all over again. Somehow, in Restorative Yoga, we give ourselves permission to feel this burden, and even to face it. This doesn't mean that we've wasted all the time spent carrying our burden. We may come to realize that our burden is not so shameful or so different from anyone else's. We may develop a sense of humor about how much we demand of ourselves and how we blame ourselves when we backslide. This helps us build perseverance and strength of character. It also helps us start to know ourselves better. We begin to experience our emotions in a way that promotes awareness and growth.

When these things happen, we can give ourselves credit for all our hard work. Yet we may also wonder: Is this the end point of our evolution? Or is there something else waiting for us on the other side of our growth?

Breath Exercise: Worrying and 1:2 Breathing

In the preceding breath exercises (at the end of chapters 1–3), you experienced three types of breath regulation. First, you observed your breath and noted its patterns. Then, you adjusted your breath to an equal inhale-to-exhale ratio. Third, you regulated your breath further by making your exhale longer than—or twice as long as—your inhale. In this exercise, you'll combine a mind-calming breathwork technique (1:2 ratio or longer exhale) with something that stimulates your mental anxiety (worrying). This exercise is more challenging than the previous three because it involves creating an anxiety pattern in the mind *while* you're using 1:2 Breathing. Balancing these two techniques can be difficult. Please make sure that you've become comfortable with the other three breathing exercises first before trying this one. If you haven't practiced them, do so first to make sure you have a stable foundation of awareness.

When you attempt Worrying and 1:2 Breathing, it's likely that your mind will worry far more if you lose your focus on the 1:2 breath ratio. If this happens to an uncomfortable degree, feel free to continue just with 1:2 Breathing, or stop the exercise and return to it later. If you're practicing 1:2 Breathing (you can even make the exhale three times longer than the inhale), you will most likely not be able to worry as intensely as you did before. If you find that you can't worry as much, that's the point of the exercise! In many ways this exercise is impossible to do correctly, because 1:2 Breathing and worrying are typically unable to coexist. In fact, 1:2 Breathing (which slows your heart rate and calms your nervous system) and worrying (which increases your heart rate and stimulates your nervous system) are for the most part incompatible. You're doing this exercise, then, to refine your awareness of how 1:2 Breathing affects the mind and nervous system quickly and effectively.

Get Your Baseline

Once again, in this exercise, you'll combine a calming (1:2 ratio) breathwork technique with something that stimulates your anxiety (worrying). First get your mental and emotional baseline: How do you feel now? Are you worried? Thinking about the future? Focused on past events? Feeling down? Take a moment to record your thoughts and feelings before you begin.

Do the Practice

Think of something that worries you or makes you angry. For this part of the exercise, keep your eyes open. Begin to think about the conflict or situation you've chosen. For the moment, don't worry about *how* you're breathing—it doesn't matter. Just spend a couple of minutes immersed in the feeling. Let your thoughts run wild, even making the situation more dramatic in your mind's eye. Now get another baseline; take your current mental and emotional "temperature." If you choose, you can also take your pulse as you did in 1:2 Breathing (page 72).

Now you're ready to begin the breathwork part. Slowly close your eyes. As you've done several times before, direct your neutral focus to your breath. Breathe in and out through your nose. Lengthen both your inhale and your exhale. See if you can increase them by a couple of counts, or seconds. Try neither to force the breath, nor to create a sense of constriction in your chest.

When your nasal breathing appears to be stable, experiment with lengthening your exhale; first let it be just one count longer than your inhale. If you breathe in for two counts, let your exhale be three counts. If you breathe in for three counts, let your exhale be four counts. See how the longer exhale feels.

If it feels comfortable, transition to an even longer exhale, letting it be double the length of your inhale. If you breathe in for two counts, exhale for four. If you breathe in for three counts, exhale for six, and so on. You can even lengthen the exhale further. For example, if you breathe in for two counts, try exhaling for five or six counts. When three to five minutes have passed, slowly open your eyes. Take your new baseline: are you still as worried or emotional as before? Note how you feel in your journal or on a piece of paper. If you wish, you can take your pulse again for comparison. Has it decreased? This is your mid-exercise baseline.

Now slowly close your eyes and resume 1:2 Breathing. When you have spent another minute with this breath ratio, think about your troublesome situation again. See whether you can attain the same level of worry or anger that existed before your breathwork. As you're doing 1:2 Breathing, if you're not as worried or stimulated, this means that you've experienced the powerful impact of breath on your mood. If you remain as worried as you were before, or still a little worried, check in with your breath; chances are that without realizing it, you lost the 1:2 breath ratio.

Feel the Difference

If you didn't attain your previous level of anxiety or anger while doing your breathwork, note that in your journal. You've just experienced firsthand the power of breath to adjust your mental state and mood. If you worried only a little bit while doing your breathing, note that as well.

If you find that you worried as much as before you started but can still practice 1:2 Breathing, be patient with the process—it'll get easier. Have compassion for your developing ability to calm your nervous system, rather than becoming convinced that none of it is working. Sometimes it takes patience, and more practice, to feel the difference.

Body Exercise: Getting to Know Restorative Yoga

The first two body-centered exercises in this book, Distinguishing between Tension and Relaxation and the Five-Minute Body

Check-in, helped you refine your body awareness. They also deepened your perception of physical discomfort (which can activate your nervous system). These exercises are preludes to the Restorative Yoga practice. If either of them felt difficult or unnatural, consider spending more time with them before moving on to this one. To feel how your body and mind respond to Restorative Yoga, you will first try Relaxation Pose (page 191), a back-bending restorative posture.

Get Your Baseline

Before practicing this exercise, check in with your body. Is your physical energy level low, medium, or high? Now notice your mind: Are your thoughts flowing at a slow, medium, or fast rate? Record your physical and mental baselines.

Do the Practice

Approach this experience in an exploratory way, especially if this is your first time practicing Restorative Yoga. Find a space where you can relax, uninterrupted, for at least five minutes. In Restorative Yoga, we reduce sensory stimulation to calm the mind and nervous system. To help with this, turn off the lights or dim them to a low setting. Practice in a quiet area. If possible, place an eye pillow or a towel over your eyes to shut out the light.

Lie down on your back with a bolster, couch cushion, or pillows under your knees. It's possible that your neck will hyperextend when you lie down on your back; if this is the case, your chin will rise into the air, and you may feel discomfort at the back of your neck. If this happens, place a folded blanket under your head for support. If you'd like more specific instructions on supporting this pose, see Relaxation Pose (page 192).

As you rest here, breathe in and out through your nose. Focus on bringing your breath to different parts of your body sequentially, as you did with the Distinguishing between Tension and Relaxation exercise (page 31). At first, try the breath ratio most natural to you. Then, if your mind feels balanced or slow, move into 1:1 Breathing.

If your mind is fast and your thoughts race, try a longer exhale or 1:2 Breathing instead. Keep directing your breath to your body, using your breath to release any tension or discomfort that you can. After five to ten minutes, slowly transition onto your side and come up to sitting.

Feel the Difference

With your eyes closed, notice the effects of this pose in your body. Does your body have more energy, but in a calm and balanced way, or is it too energized? If your body felt too energized during this exercise, don't be concerned. You may simply have a lot of energy or activity in your body. If this is the case, the forward-bending or neutral restorative poses might work better for you.

As you practiced Relaxation Pose, what happened to your mind? If your thoughts raced during the pose, don't be concerned. You may simply have anxiety in your body, and lying on your back may not be right for you. Or, you may have in your mind a dormant anxiety, which this posture simply awakened. If you notice this happening, you've taken an important step in growing your self-awareness. Mental or physical anxiety while in a back-bending posture may mean that it's best to start off your practice with forward-bending or neutral restorative postures. Record these effects in your notes to help you determine which restorative poses will be most helpful for your body and mind. You will also find a detailed list of recommendations for what to do if your mind became anxious in chapter 8 (page 187).

5

Finding Meaning in Anxiety and Depression

ERIC, A CHILDHOOD FRIEND OF MINE, WAS TWENTY-FIVE when his life first fell apart. He had just graduated with an MBA and signed on to work with a progressive new company. He bought a sky-blue BMW and purchased a penthouse condominium with a roof deck that boasted a 360-degree view of the Dallas skyline. He installed a sauna and wet bar in the basement, and his new coworkers flocked to his home for the wild parties he'd always dreamed of throwing. He bought his long-term girlfriend a gigantic diamond ring. He felt invincible, as if nothing could touch him. After a year of fast living, the company he worked for was implicated in a Ponzi scheme and Eric was one of the first to lose his job. He'd overextended himself financially and saved very little; within three months, he defaulted on his condo, and his car was next to go. "I can take this," he vowed. He moved in with Marianne, his fiancée, until he could get back on his feet. He spent nearly three hours a day in the gym, trying to maintain his appearance. To save money, he snacked on samples at Whole Foods, where he used his good looks and charm to wile seconds and thirds from the deli counter staff to cut his food costs. He continued to party hard, but on the inside, his spirits were slipping. When six months passed with no job offers, Eric's dream of getting back his old life and his old sense of invulnerability faded away. Most of his friends, attracted to his money and status, disappeared as well. Eric became morose. He stopped exercising and taking care of himself. He lay on the couch, unshowered, drinking beer and watching SportsCenter. Eventually, Marianne broke up with him, and his melancholy deepened into a full-blown depression. Eric ended up in therapy, taking two antidepressants and trying to figure out where things went wrong. "If I could just get a new job," he kept saying, "I could have my old life back."

If Eric had lived in a different society—say, with an indigenous tribe such as the !Kung Bushmen of Africa's Kalahari Desert—things might have unfolded differently. His losses and the depression that followed them might have been met with excitement. The tribal shaman, or healer, could have concluded that Eric was in the midst of a shamanic *initiation*: a process of psychic or physical suffering that precedes new understanding or rebirth, and transforms a neophyte shaman into a healer. Eric might have gone on a vision quest designed to teach him about his two selves: the one he was leaving behind and the one he was about to become. When he'd returned, the community might have held a ceremony to celebrate Eric's transition to a new identity.

Many cultures, such as the !Kung, recognize that we regularly pass from one stage of life to the next. They believe that the wisdom and integration each stage brings are often the fruits of suffering or loss. They develop rites of passage to help us transform our pain into learning. These cultures trust that the best thing to do during challenging times is to connect with ourselves as deeply as possible within the support of a community. In modern Western culture, however, rather than question the reason behind our suffering, we tend to wonder why it has to happen at all. The answer may be more metaphysical than we think: the pain, in fact, may have a hidden purpose.

Anxiety and Depression Are Opportunities in Disguise

Anxiety and depression can be dark nights of the soul, exceptionally difficult life passages that shake our foundations and threaten to break our spirit. Yet when we stay conscious through these challenging passages, we can use them to propel ourselves into healthier ways of emotional and spiritual being.

As many cultures recognize, initiations often begin with a painful experience such as anxiety, depression, physical illness, or loss. This "call to awakening," to use mythologist Joseph Campbell's term, challenges us to the depths of our being. Our suffering often strips away things such as stature, comfort, or identity that we might not voluntarily have given up. The tough part is that sometimes the pain and loss make it hard to recognize the call to awakening for what it is. Sometimes, it looks a lot like plain old suffering.

Initiations ask that we open our eyes and be present in the midst of our suffering. They ask us to trust the pain and allow it to break us open. What makes this so difficult? It's that initiations are transitional; they leave us between worlds. We enter an in-between space where our old identity is gone and we don't yet have a new one. We may wonder what will happen to us, or whether we'll be OK. During a yoga therapy session, a client anxiously asked, "If I let go of all this, will I still be myself?" She was often miserable in her old life, but the thought of a new one scared her even more.

In my work as a psychologist and yoga therapist, I've noticed several key transition times: when we're in between stages of life, jobs, partners, yoga poses, and sleeping and waking. Even the space between an exhale and an inhale (or inhale and exhale) is a transition. We may become suddenly anxious: How can we be sure we'll get to the next place intact? These transitional times are paradoxical: though often deeply unsettling, they also contain unlimited possibilities.

When a snake sheds its skin, it undergoes a temporary period of blindness. Similarly, when we slough off aspects of ourselves during transitions, we may lose our vision of who we are and where we fit in the world. What's more, we can suddenly see the filter through which we experience life—our way of interpreting what happens to us and why—for what it is. But when that filter has been distorted by anxiety and depression, we want it to change. And we can use the temporary sightlessness of transitions to develop other senses, including inner sight, or wisdom. These other senses, in turn, will change the way we filter our experience.

My students often ask me why we need these initiations simply to reach a better place. Can't we get there without the suffering? Most of the time, the answer is no—especially not if we shy away from challenges or retreat to our comfort zone. We need anxiety and depression, these emotional rites of passage, because we tend to avoid the conflict and contraction, the pain and struggle that ultimately lead to transformation. We may even prefer anxiety and depression, the devils we already know, to the devils we've yet to meet. As a client of mine once complained during a particularly trying time, "I know things are bad, but if I rock the boat, they could become unbearable!" The thing is, spiritual well-being demands a kind of sea change, a shaking up of life as we know it, that takes us out of our comfort zone and lays us open. Anxiety and depression are just this kind of sea change. But unless we understand the larger purpose of initiations, we can become stuck in anxiety and depression, unable either to go back or to transform. When this happens, we're "lost in transition."

In life, we tend to prefer structured spaces. In yoga, we tend to feel better in definable poses. On the mat, for instance, poses such as Upward Dog and Downward Dog can feel like "real" parts of our practice, but getting into and out of them can seem like empty spaces or "awareness breaks." Take the transition that occurs at the end of a restorative practice, for example. Each week, as I guide practitioners through the class, they settle in and achieve a degree of relaxation and calm. But just as the class ends, and I bring people through the slow transition up to sitting, an anxious person might pop up like a jack-in-the-box as though the transition were a waste of time. Although it's unintentional, some of the calmness developed in the practice is then lost. During life transitions, we often move from one place to the next with similar urgency, lack of awareness, or intense desire to get to the next defined space. We try to put a frame around our experience, to help us know where we are and to make life feel safe. But yoga offers us many opportunities to be present in the mind and body, even when it's uncertain, scary, or painful.

A restorative yoga practice includes many transitional openings: the interplay between the inhale and the exhale, getting into and out of a pose, the coming and going of thoughts, and the entrance and exit of feelings and sensations. The next time you encounter one of these openings, slow things down. Resist the urge to rush to the next place. Instead, work on breathing and staying present with your direct experience. Hang in there and see what emerges. At the very least, you'll start building inner trust.

The Hidden Blessing in Suffering

At times in our lives, we may encounter periods of high stress that bubble up into worry or spiral down into despair. Or we can be shadowed instead by a low-grade fear or sadness. We may even know anxiety or depression on an intimate, long-term, and serious basis. In response to our suffering we may wonder, *Why does this have to happen to me?*

We may think that our emotional pain stems from a chemical imbalance, genetic illness, difficult childhood, or just bad luck. Or we may see our patterns clearly but be unable to change them. We may try therapy, medication, support groups, holistic treatment, or work on our issues alone. The difficult life passage inaugurated by anxiety and depression may start to "stretch out" and seem indistinguishable from life itself. This makes us feel as though we've been anxious or depressed forever. We can even start to see this transitional space as a permanent reflection of who we are.

How can such difficult experiences be nourishing? When we are suffocated by depression or charged with relentless anxiety, it can seem impossible to use what's happening to us as a vehicle for evolution. But when we surrender control, we can take advantage of the hidden gifts that anxiety and depression offer us: an awakening to what's not working in our lives, an opening to the potential for growth.

Life is not static; it constantly evolves. Our cells are a good example: they mature, die, and are replaced by new cells at regular intervals. We, too, are meant to periodically slough off old aspects of ourselves so that new ones can emerge. But we can't evolve without letting go.

In 2008, I had reconstructive hip surgery for problems related to a childhood injury. Before the surgery, I contended with a lot of surprise from people: "But you're a yoga teacher," they said. "*You're* not supposed to need hip surgery." I chose to have my surgery in Belgium, where a world-renowned specialist might be able to preserve my range of motion. Not knowing what to expect, I had little choice but to surrender. I had to let go of my moment-to-moment control of my life and work back in the United States, and even of language (many of the doctors and nurses spoke either Dutch or German, which I did not). After a three-hour surgery under general anesthesia, I practiced a special breath technique in recovery that I created from combinations of yogic breathing exercises. This left me lucid, with virtually no pain. The hours passed as I listened to Mozart on my iPod and watched the sun rise, move across the sky, and then set outside my window. Surrendering not only helped me survive the experience, but opened the door to possibilities I hadn't imagined. Beginning with impromptu yoga therapy sessions with the curious medical staff at the clinic, my teaching expanded to Europe and I made some wonderful new friends. But before all this could happen, I had to relinquish control with no guarantee that things would be better.

The struggle between control and letting go can occur right on the yoga mat. In a pose that's mentally or physically difficult, we can tighten up. Let's say that we're stretching our hamstrings and encounter unexpected resistance. The mind may try to exert control and push us further into the pose to force the body to open. This struggle to open the body can, ironically, activate the nervous system and cause the body to contract and close. Recently in class, I assisted a young yoga practitioner who kept trying, throughout her practice, to compel her hips to open. As I physically and verbally guided her into the pose, I could see that she wasn't breathing, and her face was taut with effort. I could hear her berating herself under her breath. "Just breathe," I told her. "*Allow* your body to do what it already knows how to do." When she went one or two levels away from the extreme pose, she found a measure of release and flexibility. She came up after class and said, "That hit the nail on the head; pushing myself is one of my biggest issues." Difficult times in our lives work in much the same way. It's natural to want to force change, to urge ourselves into the next space that the mind wants us to occupy. And it's human nature to contract and tense up. I know; I've been there myself. But when we struggle against the web of resistance that binds us, it simply grows tighter.

Frequently, someone will come to my restorative class with the rounded shoulders and collapsed chest of depression. Gung ho to change this pattern, she may drape her body over a high rise of props designed to get her heart area to open. To compensate for this massive opening, her shoulders and chest have to round and collapse further, and her neck must hyperextend. She may be in intense discomfort, but her mind believes that this extreme move- ment is the *only way* to open her chest and shoulders. No pain, no gain, she likely thinks. The problem here is that this forced open- ing creates muscular tension, which puts the nervous system into overdrive. This, together with the extra contraction in her shoul- ders, reinforces the very pattern she wishes to change. Ironically, when we lower the height of her bolster and add extra support to her shoulders, we *suggest* the opening rather than compel it. With support, we put the shoulders, chest, and upper back in a position to relax and open up a little: from point A to point D. They can then receive the breath. When they do, the mind can expand to receive compassion, and perhaps even learn how to partner with the body to create change.

Restorative Yoga doesn't guarantee an immediate end to our pain. But its combination of physical relaxation and mental alert- ness helps us notice where we are holding on. We can be present with the holding and breathe into it. Our muscles can receive the breath and begin to relax. This also helps the mind to loosen its iron grip on our experience. When it does, it hangs on less tightly to anxiety and depression. This creates a deep listening space where presence can rush in and fill us.

The practices in this book help us detect and feel physical tight- ness, mental worry or sadness, or general emotional pain. They offer us the physical and mental support to tolerate, breathe through, and liberate these patterns. This allows us to move beyond the patterns, and even to ask questions of our anxiety and depression. Five questions, in particular, offer deep spiritual growth. These questions approach the essence of who we are and what we're meant to do with our lives. They help us transform anxiety and depression from dark nights of the soul into the dawning of a more profound connection with our deepest self. With all five essential questions, our task is to inquire without looking for an immediate answer. The answer most often emerges over time, when we're not forcing it to arrive.

Essential Question 1: What Is My Anxiety or Depression Trying to Teach Me?

When anxiety and depression open a window into a world of new possibility, as they did for my childhood friend Eric, you're meant to climb through that window. You're not supposed to get your old life back; you're expected to begin a new one. The first essential question in creating a new life is: *What is my anxiety or depression trying to teach me?* In the midst of a challenging time, this is a hard question to ask.

Petra, a yoga therapy client, never thought that her carefully constructed world would ever crumble. She knew what she wanted out of life: to make partner at her law firm by the age of thirty-two. Since childhood, she'd set stunningly high standards for herself. She'd been class president in grade school, captain of the debate team and class valedictorian in high school, student union president and varsity swim team captain in college, and editor of the law review in law school. Petra was driven to construct an invincible exterior that she could display to the world. She did this through her legal conquests, becoming what she jokingly termed a "corporate piranha." There were numerous casualties: her job devoured friendships, love relationships, even the warmth she had with her parents and sister. Yet the further upstream she swam, the less she seemed to care.

Then, just as Petra turned thirty-two, a colleague who'd joined the firm two years after she did received a promotion. Petra began to unravel. She became convinced that the managing partner thought her incompetent. She increased her work hours and brought in more cases than anyone else in her firm; she forced her secretary to work seventy-five hours a week just to keep up. But she paid the price. She developed anxiety and insomnia; her brain just refused to "turn off." She had several episodes of heart palpitations and chest pain so severe that she feared she was having a heart attack. Several times, she was hospitalized for observation; while there, she relentlessly text-messaged her colleagues and terrorized the nurses for moving too slowly. When I first met her, Petra seemed invulnerable and made of stone; she rarely showed emotion. When she told me of her mother's slow death from lung cancer, she clenched her jaw as though she were angry. Yet I could see that underneath her rock-hard exterior a more vulnerable, intuitive self was hiding.

What might Petra's anxiety have to teach her? When I asked her, she admitted to a nagging feeling that not making partner was a sign. She hadn't wanted to contemplate this before because it would challenge her single-pointed focus on success. Perhaps, she said, she needed to slow down and take stock of her life. Recently, she'd felt a "vat of loneliness and sorrow" welling up from within. She hoped that yoga would bring her more in touch with her body and her feelings. Despite her natural impatience, she was willing to turn to contemplative and therapeutic yoga practices until the answers to her questions revealed themselves. Like Petra, you can use your emotional pain as an opportunity for self-study. What might *your* anxiety or depression have to teach you? And how might your life change if you asked?

Essential Question 2: What Is the Balance between
My Inner and Outer Awareness?

Anxiety and depression are messengers; they tell us of an imbalance between our connection to the outer world and the inner self. A high level of sensory stimulation from the outer world (think iPods, e-mail, television, and even our interactions with others) puts the nervous system into overdrive. When we reduce sensory stimulation and draw inward, the nervous system calms. Then we can connect with parts of ourselves that often lie buried under expectations, obligations, or self-doubt. We can also use inner awareness to ground ourselves and keep from giving our power away or centering ourselves in others' experience to the exclusion of our own. When we're too outwardly focused, we're ungrounded, and typically more anxious. But if we're too inwardly focused, we can become withdrawn, disconnected, and usually more depressed. Optimal awareness is balanced between the inner and outer worlds. So the second essential question to ask in the midst of anxiety or depression is: *What is the balance between my inner and outer awareness?* Let's delve more deeply into the interplay between these two kinds of awareness, and see how it relates to emotional balance.

Inner awareness is every bit as important to yoga as breathwork. Like breathwork (pranayama), inner awareness is given its own category of practice (*pratyahara*). Pratyahara, an inner awareness or the drawing inward of the senses, is one of the primary limbs of yoga. Pratyahara has direct bearing on the balance of our nervous system. When we use inner awareness in a balanced and skillful way, we equilibrate our nervous system and our emotions. When we don't, we contribute to emotional imbalance. So what happens to our pratyahara when we experience anxiety and depression?

Anxiety wires the nervous system to focus extensively on the outer world. With a hyperalert nervous system, we work overtime to track every nuance in our environment. We try to anticipate and manage the steady stream of demands placed on us. This uninterrupted, periscope-like vigilance means that we can't risk going inward for fear that something threatening will catch us by surprise. It can feel as though the outer world is the only thing we *can* control (an illusion, of course) and that the inner world is unknown, an ocean of possibility for danger. When Derek, one of my clients, first began practicing pratyahara (in the form of the Five-Minute Body Check-in, page 50), he realized something about himself. Anxiety, he said, had drawn his focus outward for so long that he felt divorced from his inner self. If you suffer from anxiety, like Derek, you will benefit from using the Anxiety-Balancing Practice in chapter 8 of this book to help train your awareness inward.

It's not that we shouldn't look outward at all. But as a culture, we do so a lot already. Every class I teach begins with a check-in, in meditation form, to start the process of tuning in. In each check-in, we disengage from the outer world and "drop in" to the inner one. People who aren't used to looking inward or who would rather "get moving" can have a harder time of it. They can easily become distracted by a sudden need to fix their hair, go to the bathroom, or sneak a look at their cell phone one last time. Once, during an opening meditation, one of my students focused with a look of great interest and intensity at something just behind my head. I turned to look too, wondering what might be happening, only to find a squirrel cavorting in the elm outside. We all laughed together and used the term *squirrel mind* that day to capture (with humor) how easily we can get distracted from our inner awareness. Yet this inner gaze is present in every aspect of yoga: breathing, active postures, restorative postures, and meditation.

Depression tinges our focus in a different way than anxiety. In depression, we frequently struggle to move awareness away from our negative and self-defeating inner worlds. It's as though we are flooded by thought, sensation, and emotion. We can become lost within an inner labyrinth of negativity, with little compassion to guide us. We may resist emerging for fear we'll encounter the same sort of criticism we experience on the inside. Even though this can seem like looking inward, it's not; in depression, a relentless self-focus can permeate pratyahara. We may avoid a true connection with others and with the world. Faye, a longtime student of mine, focused her awareness inward, but exclusively on painful physical and emotional sensations. Her depression left her without the energy to connect with her family and friends. Since Faye never made an effort to reach out to them, they understandably experienced her depression as selfishness and a lack of desire to communicate. Focusing some of her energy on connecting with others would help to balance Faye's inner and outer awareness. If you suffer from depression, like Faye, you can benefit from the Depression-Lifting Practice in chapter 9. You'll also benefit from asking Essential Question 3, which gets at the nature of pratyahara, of what it looks like when you draw your attention inward.

Balancing anxiety and depression requires that we cultivate our inner world in a healthy way. We can spend time focusing on the breath. We can engage in direct experience of the body while moving in an active practice or relaxing in a restorative one. We can go deeply into internal sensations such as anxiety, hunger, sadness, even muscular tightness or discomfort, but not so deeply that we become engulfed by them.

Drawing awareness inward *in a healthy way* is essential to shifting our emotional patterns. It guides us in choosing the best interventions for our emotional state. It helps us to notice and integrate the effects of what we practice. It enables us to watch our emotional patterns in action. It makes *us*, rather than a doctor, psychologist, or healer, the emotional electrician and rewiring expert. This may be scary, perhaps, but it's ultimately empowering.

At the beginning of my yoga workshops, I always share with participants that compassionate, yet neutral observation of the self is one of our most important interventions in balancing anxiety and depression. They look almost disappointed, as if to say, "But that's so *ordinary*!" Unglamorous though it may seem, the inner gaze of pratyahara is as powerful as any of yoga's subtle tools. It strengthens our ability to feel, process, and contain our emotions, which is of great benefit in anxiety and depression. Yet it's not just a matter of *whether* we look inward. The third essential question involves *how* we do so.

Essential Question 3: What Is the Quality of My Inner Gaze?

The act of tuning in asks that we face our painful thoughts and emotions head-on. Looking inside can feel intolerable if we habitually look inward with a *hardness*, a quality of meanness or judgment. So the third essential question for us to ask of our anxiety and depression is: *What is the quality of my inner gaze?* In other words, what is the quality with which I look at myself and my "stuff"?

Often in yoga class, a student will tell me (always in an attempt to be helpful), "My hips are bad," or "I'm not very flexible," or even "I'm bad at yoga." Building on the belief that the body is flawed in some way, our mind begins to critique itself: it sees us as useless, unworthy, or out of control. From here, it takes very little to conclude that our *inner self* is bad or inflexible. The tendency to judge the things we say or do, how we look, even our feelings, is human. At the same time, it is dehumanizing. It harms the inner self.

Recently, one of my colleagues brought her six-year-old daughter, Lila, to class. Although Lila was initially shy and played quietly on her mat, she soon became engaged in the class. She suggested poses for me to teach, and practiced them on her mat along with everyone else. Within a short period of time, to the delight of the class, Lila came up to the front of the room to teach Eagle Pose, Boat Pose, and Tortoise Pose. She even discussed the benefits of Tortoise Pose, assuring the class that one minute in the pose would make them feel as though they'd slept for eight hours. Lila was completely in her element, immersed in what she was doing without worrying about how she looked or what people would think. Her inner magic infected the class, and everyone left with smiles on their faces.

As very young children, we naturally trusted the deepest self. Without even thinking, we connected with it. Children's characteristic self-trust helps grace to flourish and extend into the body, which is why most young children have excellent posture. Somewhere along the line, as our child selves grow older, we learn that approval comes mostly when we perform well by someone else's standards. We start to expend time and energy attempting to figure out those standards. We experience how disappointing others brings disapproval, potential rejection, and even abandonment. So, many of us relinquish our self-trust and creativity little by little in favor of the drive to be good. We internalize others' judgments until they become our own.

This self-judgment becomes especially poignant every year in my teacher-training class. In their assisting module, teachers-in-training learn how to adjust practitioners' poses. Each year, I warn the class what might happen. I tell them that for some, a pattern of needing to "get it right" might take over. Still, it catches them by surprise. Suddenly, the joy of helping another student deepen a posture or awaken a "sleeping" part of the body can fade, only to be replaced by intense performance anxiety. Although the practitioners' bodies communicate clearly what adjustments are needed, some of the teachers-in-training stop looking and really *seeing* the bodies in front of them. They've already moved into their heads, where the critical self lives. Then, they accelerate into what we call "freak-out mode," where the mind worries about their performance. Inevitably, because their nervous systems are buzzing with anxiety, their breathing becomes shallow. They abandon all direct experience in their bodies, and cease being present with the bodies of the students they're trying to help. Because of all this, they practice the assist incorrectly. When this happens, they usually know that the assist has missed the boat. The inner critic uses this as food for negative thinking, and the cycle of self-judgment continues.

This struggle is such a touching one for me to witness. When the inner critic dominates, the teachers-in-training can't access their own wisdom and ability; they can't see themselves or others. If they dissociate, the struggle can "dog" them for months, even for the remainder of the training. But if they can stay present, breathe, and keep their consciousness rooted in their bodies in the midst of this struggle, the pattern changes dramatically.

This sort of self-judgment is hardly confined to yoga teacher training. It has grown so prevalent today that the concept of compassion toward the self has become an official category in psychotherapy. How might self-judgment or self-compassion play out in your life? In what situations do you go into "negative mind" and lose touch with your innate intelligence? The next time it happens, try to remain present and focused in your body, and keep breathing fully and deeply. See if that helps bring you back to yourself.

Just as we learned the harsh quality of our inner gaze, we can *unlearn* it. Through compassionate, nonjudgmental observation in our yoga practice, we can soften our inner gaze. When we stop judging ourselves (or browbeating ourselves to be less anxious or depressed), we discover something interesting. The mind, body, and nervous system have a natural sense of our true, healthy emotional set point. They already know how to make us feel better. We just need to stop thwarting them with negative thoughts and fears. Then their natural ability to balance us can kick in.

Therapeutic yoga's relaxation of the body, regulation of the breath, and alert observation of the mind form a potent combination that helps us gaze inward without judgment. When we're really present, we don't need to fix what we see. We don't feel the urge to be somewhere other than where we are. We don't want to be someone other than who we are. At the very least we need, feel, or want these things a little less. Our self-observation is free to take on a measure of compassion. This feeds the next element of spiritual awareness: figuring out who we really are, deep down.

Essential Question 4: Who Am I Not?

The fourth essential question—*Who am I not?*—might seem a little backward at first. Why not just ask, "Who am I?"

When we're young, just as we have great posture, we also know who we are. This inner knowledge helps us feel and express our emotions with exuberance. It enables us to choose or discard professions (such as firefighter, fairy, or race-car driver) with guiltless ease. Even more, it lets these budding personalities (the outer part of us) stay close to our deepest self (the inner part). And then we become self-conscious. Perhaps we have painful experiences: A teacher doesn't "see" us. A group of children make fun of us. A parent criticizes our creative impulses. We have good reasons for separating from our deepest self. We hide it to protect it from harm. We start to cloak it in layers. Eventually, we may hide this self so well that even we can't find it anymore. Sometimes, we forget it ever existed.

Once we've learned the art of hiding the deepest self, the personality also begins to suffer. We may quell our naturally rebellious instincts in favor of becoming the good girl we believe our parents need us to be. We may bury our love for composing country music to be a doctor like our father and his father before him. We can set aside the dream of playing baseball because "girls don't do that." We might suppress our natural urge to hug people when it got us into trouble at puberty. We live more in the persona, the self that's safe to show others, than anywhere else. Eventually, we may feel we *are* that persona. The question "Who am I not?" means we get to peel those layers away, one by one, until we reach the tart or juicy center of who we *are*. Though painful, anxiety and depression can strip away layers of this persona, unveiling to us our more essential and abiding qualities.

The Yoga Sutras, one of classical yoga's seminal texts, implicates this confusion between the deepest self and the outermost personality as the cause of all suffering. Sutra 2.17 states that the cause of pain is our identification of the self with the fluctuations of our personality and our emotional states. This sutra suggests that the root of all suffering is a mental error: The mind confuses our deepest parts (or essence) with our perceptions (or filter). What are these perceptions? We identify with our bodies, emotions, experiences, interactions, hopes, thoughts, and dreams. And all these things *change*. Yoga's word for everything that changes is *prakriti*. The only thing that doesn't change is the spirit, or deepest self. What does all this have to do with anxiety and depression? The more our thoughts, physical states, emotions, and behaviors change, and it's in their nature to do so on a moment-by-moment basis, the more our sense of self can become unstable.

Take, as an example, the body in yoga. A pose that feels difficult now—perhaps because our hips are tight today—simply feels difficult *right now*. It's not a sign that our hips are "bad," or that we're "inflexible" or "inept," as I so often hear in class. Through the regular practice of yoga, we come to understand that the pose may not feel the same tomorrow or next week. Then, we're not "rocked" by what we notice. We don't get caught up in it or attach great meaning to it.

Let's see how this works with the breath. Inhale, and then breathe out all your oxygen. Don't inhale again just yet. What happens? Most likely, within less than a minute, this state of holding your breath will end; your inhale will have to take over and you'll breathe again. That's just the way your breath works. Now inhale, and when you've inhaled as much as you can, hold your breath. Don't exhale just yet. . . . Within a matter of seconds, you'll have to breathe out. You do this without thinking, countless times a day. But because you're not focused on your breath, you're less likely to receive the lesson it offers. The inhale and exhale, *like everything else including thoughts, emotions, and states of mind,* are temporary. They come and they go. Yoga brings your focus to your breath and body, whether the body is still or moving. This gives you a firsthand, embodied experience of how short-lived and changeable your mind and emotions really are.

These fluctuations help us begin to recognize that we are *not* our bodies. We are *not* our emotions, experiences, or thoughts. Discomfort comes and goes. Comfort comes and goes. Anxiety and depression also fluctuate; they, too, are temporary states of being. As we observe anxiety and depression coming and going, we come to realize that we are not anxiety or depression. We start to trust that although worry or sadness may feel challenging right now, it won't *always* feel that way. The world won't feel dangerous forever. We won't feel like a loser permanently. Our anxiety or low self-esteem may not be there tomorrow or next week unless, of course, we keep feeding it. No doubt you've read this somewhere or heard it from someone you trust, and maybe even believe it to be true. While your mind may believe it, however, your body may not have experienced its truth directly. This is where yoga can help.

Once you realize that your anxiety and depression are *not* you, something else happens. You develop an understanding of all the things that ebb and flow and change, of all the things that you are *not.* You then can begin to inquire into the parts of you that don't change, into who you truly *are.* When you gaze inward, your outer sight becomes a deep, internal sight; your outer hearing becomes a deep, internal listening. The closer you get to connecting with your own true nature, the more your mind, body, and spirit align.

Essential Question 5: How Do I Relate to the World?

In anxiety and depression, we may have bought into the idea that we *are* the sum of our experiences of worry or sorrow. As a result, we may also have seen the world as a threatening place, or as a place full of rejection and loss. When we peel away the layers of who we are *not* and begin to sense what and who we are, something wonderful happens. These inner changes reflect into our outer life, changing the way we filter our experience of others and of the world. The fifth essential question is: *How do I relate to the world?*

When we learn to observe and not cling to the changing parts of ourselves (the worry, sadness, or feelings of inadequacy), we appreciate and honor the intrinsic qualities of our own spirit. Then we start to do the same with others. Yoga reveals to us not only our deepest self but others' deepest selves. I like to think of this as "soul seeing." Recently, during a session, a longtime client marveled at how different she felt during yoga. "No one sees this side of me," she said, "but you." She tried to explain what was so different and why she felt reluctant to let others see her clearly. "I just feel *more like me*," she said. This isn't New Age, airy-fairy stuff; it's real. In the practice of yoga, we encounter ourselves. When we accept our emotions and our inner nature, we can become more forgiving of others' shortcomings, real or imagined. We're less overcome by Sudden Repulsion Syndrome (which is, in the end, a turning outward of our own self-judgment). We don't need to expend effort to do this. It just seems to happen as a natural outgrowth of our practice.

At the very least, this benefits our emotional interactions with others. We go with the flow and begin to see emotions (others' and our own) not as enemies to fight but as changing interactions in our everyday, shifting landscape. Say that you feel betrayed by a good friend. You notice and experience this feeling: *Look at this feeling of betrayal that's arising; it's really intense.* You differentiate it from who you are: *This feeling of betrayal is not me; I am not betrayal. This is just a feeling and it will pass in a while.* You breathe it in and breathe it out: *I let go of this feeling that is not me.* When you do this, you come to react less strongly when others draw their emotional weapons. Rather than preparing to counterattack, you move a little to the side, and their anger misfires. It doesn't hit you head-on. Your aggressive mental dialogues stay quieter. You're better able to respond with compassion. This creates more harmonious interactions, a more balanced emotional world. You see the fault lines in others, just as you see them in yourself. When viewed through the perspective of yoga, these fault lines are affecting, even endearing. The urge to crush them like a cockroach underfoot begins to subside.

When we take the time to question anxiety and depression, we are rewarded by learning and growth. Even if we simply chose to live and grow in solitude, it would be worth our hard work and focus. Yet emotional balance and the spiritual lessons that lie beyond it become more meaningful in relation to our social world. Here, the rewards of emotional balance transcend our valid self-interest. They enrich the entire social ecosystem in which we live.

Becoming Shamans

When we go through an initiation of anxiety or depression, we have a rebirth of sorts. We become a new version of ourselves. This neophyte self has a rawness, a vulnerability. Inevitably, it will have to face yet another firing squad of outer layers (of personality) that try to shoot it down or scare it into hiding. When we've lived through this at least once, however, we're the wiser for it. And we have an array of therapeutic yoga tools that can shepherd us through it again.

When I teach at yoga conferences, the contrast between the quest for the deep self and the connection to the outermost self is illustrated in dramatic fashion. At the hotel or conference center, classes that promise relief for anxiety or depression, a more profound connection with yoga philosophy, or a stronger core body are sandwiched in next to the "yoga marketplace." The deep practice of yoga is juxtaposed against companies offering pants cleverly designed to make your butt look good and nutritionals claiming to offer you instant inner calm. The true work of steering your way through this paradox always lies with the practice itself. As Pattabhi Jois, the founder of Ashtanga Yoga, used to say, "Do your practice, and all is coming."

The suffering, death, and symbolic rebirth of initiations are mirrored within our own bodies. For example, the immune system has an extraordinary memory. It learns the complex codes of all the viruses, fungi, and bacteria we encounter. Once we've battled a foreign invader, our immune system can recall it. If we come across that pathogen again, it even remembers with astonishing accuracy the precise code that triggers its destruction.

The spiritual self has an equal capacity to remember. The shamanic tradition believes that any spirit (such as a painful illness,

memory, or experience) that played a role in cleaving us open becomes etched into our cellular memory. We can then heal all illnesses that this demon has played a part in causing. At the very
least, when we use anxiety and depression mindfully once, they
won't break us down the same way next time. And something else
happens when we make it through these dark passages of pain: we
build faith in ourselves. Create a reservoir of energy that we can
draw from whenever we need to.

My father died suddenly, shortly after his eighty-sixth birthday.
Over the final six years of his life, yoga drew us even closer together.
Beginning with the yoga book that he gave me on my eighteenth
birthday, we shared the language and practices of yoga. He even
began to enjoy Indian chanting concerts, and helped out at several
yoga studio celebrations. Beyond that, we shared the bond of mutual
transformation. Even Dad's transition from this life to the next was
infused with yoga. On the day he died, my brother and sister and I
held him and breathed with him in the ICU at Beth Israel Deacon-
ess Medical Center in Boston. Three of his best friends surrounded
his bed, and a cousin played his favorite cello concerto. Breathing
with him, our heads touching, I felt his struggle toward death. I also
experienced the long wave of peace that entered his body, the deep
exhale that signaled his final surrender. At the time, my heartache
was so profound that I doubted I could practice yoga. Yet the first
time on my mat, a day or two after his death, I was surprised by
the wellspring of energy—what yogis call *prana*—that awaited me.
The prana that I'd put into my practice over the years nourished me
when my own life force was low. Losing my father was an initiation
in itself. Remnants of the experience still remain, such as the occasional closing of a fist around my heart when a memory strikes me
a certain way. Yet his loss gives me many gifts as well.

Although I remain dedicated to helping people achieve emotional balance, my heart also lies with its spiritual expression in
the world. Our suffering has many faces, yet one root: separation
from the deepest self, or spirit. The essence of the word *yoga* is
union, and the practice of yoga unites the mind and body with the
deepest self.

We can emerge from our own suffering with an embodied understanding of the universality of emotional pain. We can realize that we are not alone. This is not only because we've discovered a connection to our deepest self. It's also because we've participated in the collective experience of suffering and death, of illumination and rebirth. We've shared in the goal of yoga: the unity of minds, bodies, and spirits into one mind, one body, and one spirit.

 ## Breath Exercise: Going with the Flow of Emotions

The two exercises that follow are more emotionally complex than the exercises in chapters 1–4 of this book. For this reason, you may want to practice your Restorative Yoga sequences ten times or more before giving these a try. If either exercise in this section feels uncomfortable, feel free to stop and return to it another time.

You can practice the following yoga technique with any of the breath exercises you've tried so far: Getting to Know Your Breath, 1:1 Breathing, or 1:2 Breathing. You can also choose to practice it while in a Restorative Yoga posture (choose Relaxation Pose [pages 185 and 191] if that worked for you before, or select your favorite restorative pose). This exercise works best when you're emotionally "stirred up," or in the grip of an emotional reaction. If at first you find it difficult to practice while feeling emotions, you can also try it in the midst of a milder emotional reaction. Then, in time, you can work your way up to a stronger emotional reaction.

Get Your Baseline

Take a moment to note how you are feeling physically and emotionally. Briefly write down any observations in your journal.

Do the Practice

Start by closing your eyes and beginning the transition to inner awareness, as you've done many times in the previous exercises. Bring your attention to your breath and lengthen both your inhale and your exhale. Use the breath ratio that has worked best for you (either 1:2 Breathing, if you are mentally stirred up, or 1:1 Breathing, if your mind feels more balanced and calm).

Step 1: Noticing. Notice the emotions surging through you. For the purpose of this exercise, pick just one emotion at a time to work with. You can go through this process with as many emotions as you like. If you can, name the emotion; you can call it sadness, fear, shame, anxiety, anger, or something else that resonates for you. If it's difficult to identify the emotion you feel today, simply call it "discomfort." As you breathe in and out through your nose, say to yourself something like, "I notice this feeling of sadness (or discomfort or whatever you are feeling). It's pretty strong today." Then note where you feel it and what it feels like, such as, "I feel it in my chest; it's like a fist closing around my heart."

Step 2: Differentiating. Continue to watch the emotion that's caught hold of you. If you can—that is, if it's comfortable for you—change your breath ratio. Try lengthening your exhale so it's just a count or two longer than your inhale. If this is stressful, return to the breath you used in step 1. Now you're ready to begin the process of differentiation. Say to yourself, "I notice this feeling of sadness (or whatever feeling you've chosen to work with). It's just a feeling; it's not me." Repeat to yourself, either out loud or in your mind, "I am not the sadness; the sadness is not me," or, "This is just a feeling, and it will pass."

Step 3: Releasing. Continue with your initial breath ratio. Or if you wish, use a longer exhale or double the length of your exhale. After several minutes of breathing, visualize yourself on a football field. Imagine your sadness or anger as a friendly opponent. Watch it charge in to tackle you and bring you down. Just as it approaches, dodge to the side a little bit. Your sadness or anger will zip past you and evaporate into the air. Watch it form into that feeling again and circle around for another pass. You have infinite patience; you can do this no matter how many passes it makes at you.

Let it approach again; sidestep it once more. Say to yourself something like, "I let go of this sadness that is not me," and "I choose to let it move around (or through) me." You can repeat this as many times as you like until you feel an appreciation for the dance of your emotions appearing, fading, and returning back to you. Feel how your emotions come and go. When you're ready, send your emotion into the air. Let it fly in a high, lazy arc, sunlight glinting off its helmet, out over the field. Watch it disappear into the clouds, where it becomes your favorite bird—real or fictional.

As you continue to breathe for several minutes, imagine your emotion flying above cloud level. See it join other migrations of feelings that are coming and going across the sky.

Feel the Difference

When you slowly transition onto your side and come up to sitting, notice whether you feel different. Is your mind calmer and centered? Or still racing around? How about your body? If it's hard to get this technique to work immediately, stick with it. Like the other exercises in this book, it takes time and practice to set new patterns. Patience and self-compassion ensure that time is on your side.

Body Exercise: Inhabiting Your Body with Kindness

In this exercise, you'll build on the foundation of comfort and support that you created in the four previous body awareness exercises: Distinguishing between Tension and Relaxation, the Five-Minute Body Check-in, Going Up the Stairs Backward, and Getting to Know Restorative Yoga. If you've practiced these earlier exercises, you are ready for a deeper check-in. If you haven't yet done so, it's best to try them before this one.

In the first four body awareness exercises, you began to develop the ability to look inward and inhabit your body. Now it's time to add another element to your check-in: getting in touch with the quality or "attitude" of your inner gaze, the way in which you look inward. You can choose to practice this while you relax in a Restorative Yoga pose such as Relaxation Pose (see pages 185 and 191 for instructions).

Here, you'll infuse your check-in with comfort, support, relaxation, and a quality of kindness often missing in anxiety and depression patterns. If you have trouble summoning that level of kindness, don't worry; even if self-compassion has been in short supply for you lately, you'll find it—it may just take a little time.

Get Your Baseline

Go to your quiet space where you can practice uninterrupted for ten to fifteen minutes. When you get your baseline, observe the quality of your inner gaze, your looking inward. You can use this quality as a diagnostic tool. Does your gaze focus on what's around you or race from one thing to the next, as it would in anxiety? Or does it get lost in the inner criticism and negative dialogue that's characteristic of depression?

Allow an intention for your practice to rise to the surface of your awareness. Today, let your intention, and your practice, be imbued with gentleness and compassion. Then take a moment to get a baseline for how you feel today. If you feel anxious, give yourself a number on a 1–10 scale, with "10" being extremely anxious and "1" being not at all anxious. Also, note the level of ease and comfort in your body. If it helps, you can use your 1–10 scale again here. This brief check-in resembles the kind of check-in that you'd do each time you do a restorative practice.

Do the Practice

Now you're ready to begin. Keep in mind that slow and fluid transitions benefit both anxiety and depression, and make the most of every transition. Even the slowness and care with which you set up your support is important. Sit comfortably with your legs crossed, with several inches of elevation (a bolster, pillows, or blanket) under your sitting bones. Add pillows under your thighs to support your knees if they relax better with support. Adopt any modifications necessary for your comfort. You can extend your legs, prop your back up against a wall, or lie on your back with your knees bent.

Transition your eyelids slowly to closed. Allow the closing of your eyes to signal your mind and body that you are moving from *outer* awareness to a deep, internal awareness. If your mind wanders or your sensory awareness moves outward, that's natural; it's a long-held habit and takes practice to change. Notice it with a sense of compassion and shift your awareness back inward.

Breathe slowly, in and out through your nose. Direct your breath to your eyes. As you've done before, let your eyeballs relax and move inward, dropping a little toward your heart. Feel how your outer sight slowly becomes inner sight, or *in*sight. Let your ears also begin to draw inward, coming to join your eyes at your heart. Feel how your outer hearing transforms into a deep, internal listening. Even if you can't immediately feel your deepest self, the inner movement of awareness helps you make contact and begin to listen to its voice. Just cultivate compassion in whatever way you can.

Continue to draw your attention inward and focus on your body. Notice any discomfort or tension there. Let go of any judgment that arises in response to this discomfort. Instead, just bring your breath to that part of the body. Breathe in compassion and nonjudgment. Notice what is happening right now—perhaps together, your compassion and your breath can soften that part of your body.

As you inhale, imagine that you're drawing in life force, positive energy, faith, and hope. As you exhale, imagine that you're releasing judgment, negativity, doubt, and despair. You are building a reservoir of compassion and kindness. Continue to observe your body for the next couple of minutes. Note any physical sensations such as hunger, thirst, comfort, unease, energy, or fatigue. Observe what you are noticing without needing to get caught up in it; just notice it and then let go.

Now focus once more on your breath. Continue to breathe slowly in and out through your nose. Bring your awareness to your mind, where your thoughts come from. As you continue to breathe, notice the thoughts that pass through your awareness. What quality do they have? Are they distracting? Negative? Hopeful? How fast are your thoughts coming? Just notice without judgment. If you're preoccupied and obsessing over something, notice that too. You can assign a speed to your thoughts, with "10" representing racing thoughts that are coming almost faster than you can handle and "1" being slow, "molasses-like" thinking.

Look at the quality of your inner gaze. If you find yourself in the midst of critical self-evaluation, try to lengthen both your inhale and your exhale. Release some of the self-critical quality as you breathe out. Remember that lack of self-compassion feeds anxiety and depression; it helps keep them alive. You *can* unlearn the way you've become used to evaluating yourself, just as you can learn to bring more self-compassion and kindness to what you see in yourself.

Bring your focus back to your breath; breathe in and out through your nose. Next, allow your awareness to travel into your emotions. Note the tone of your emotional self today: Are you feeling optimistic? Anxious? Sad? Stressed? Just notice, without needing to become attached to what you are noticing in any way. Notice and let it go. You can even ask the question, "What does this emotion have to teach me?" Just ask, without needing an answer.

Feel the Difference

You've now traveled into your body, your mind, and your emotional self. Take a few minutes to breathe quietly, still keeping your focus linked to your breath. When you're ready to begin the transition out of your check-in, let your awareness travel a little closer to the surface: somewhere between inner sight and outer sight, inner hearing and outer hearing. Take a moment to check back in with your body, your mind, and your emotions. Observe any changes or shifts that have occurred. Stay impartial, if possible, when noticing these shifts.

When you're ready, gently transition your eyes to open. You may, if you wish, record in your notebook any observations from your check-in. Do you notice a difference, however small, after this exercise? Has practicing self-compassion and kindness lessened your depression or anxiety a bit? Training your attention inward, *with kindness*, is one of the most effective ways to interrupt an anxiety or depression pattern. Remember that it takes repeated practice, over time, to create lasting change in your patterns.

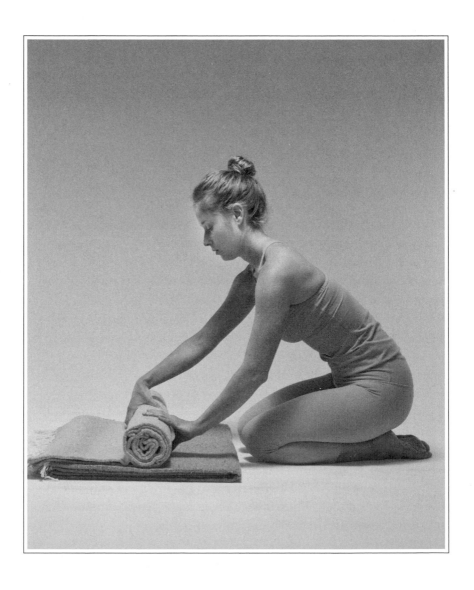

PART TWO

Breathwork and Restorative Yoga

6

What's Your Emotional Type?

USUALLY, WHEN PHYSICAL PAIN OR ILLNESS FIRST APPEARS, we spend time and effort cataloging our symptoms. Then we visit a doctor and describe how we feel. The doctor's responsibility is to make a diagnosis and offer treatment. With anxiety and depression, however, the doctor's task becomes more complex. In the diagnostic guidelines that doctors use, symptoms of anxiety and depression can overlap: Signs of anxiety can occur in depression, and elements of depression can seep into anxiety. How can the doctor accurately distinguish one from the other?

As we discussed in chapter 1, the Integrative Yoga Therapeutics system recognizes this challenge. It answers it by classifying symptoms of anxiety and depression into two categories: physical and mental. This classification then gives rise to four primary types of emotional imbalance. The first two are straightforward: anxiety in both body and mind, and depression in both body and mind. The last two types involve mixtures of anxiety and depression: one combines depression in the body with anxiety in the mind, and the other blends anxiety in the body with depression in the mind.

This chapter offers a description of each of the emotional types; as you read them, you can determine which type most closely matches your mind and body. Then, you'll choose the practice that fits your emotional type. This enables you to become an "emotional detective" and take control of your own healing. Through particular combinations of breathwork and Restorative Yoga, you can address one kind of symptom in your body, and the same—or a different— kind of symptom in your mind. On days when your physical energy is depressed but your thoughts are anxious, you can create a practice that energizes your body but keeps your mind more balanced and calm, and vice versa. In this way, therapeutic yoga is a powerful practice for people who suffer from anxiety or depression alone, from a mixture of the two, or from fluctuations between anxiety and depression. As you read through the descriptions here, it might be useful to have a pen and paper handy so you can take notes and consider which scenario best describes your experience. This helps you hone your skills as an emotional detective. For extra help with self-diagnosis and building awareness, try the Five-Minute Body Check-in (page 50). As you become more adept at tracking your physical and emotional symptoms, you can tailor your practice to your changing needs.

If you're not sure which type of emotional balance best describes you, try each of the four practices in chapters 8–10 and feel which one resonates the most. Remember that ultimately, *you* have the power to know yourself better, to become your own yoga therapist, no matter how difficult it might seem at first.

Let's take some time to explore the four types of emotional imbalance in greater depth. We'll start first with the two straightforward types.

Emotional Type 1:
Anxious Body/Anxious Mind

The Anxious Body/Anxious Mind form of emotional imbalance means that you have anxiety in both your body and your mind. Rob, one of my longtime yoga students, is a great example. Rob is constantly on the go, rarely stopping to rest or take stock of his surroundings. A computer programmer by trade, he obsessively searches the Internet, checks e-mail, or updates his Facebook page, even when he's at work or on a lunch break. His fidgetiness sets his friends on edge, and he moves so rapidly that he appears frenzied and less graceful than he really is. Nicknamed "the Energizer" because his friends so seldom see his "battery" wear down, Rob has a habit of jiggling his right knee with such intensity that it threatens to topple over the table at mealtimes. He eats so fast that he finishes his food long before his companions. He leaves behind a litter of crumbs, complains of an upset stomach, and mournfully badgers his friends by asking, "Why did you let me eat all that?" His friends have to guard their plates from Rob's restless scavenging of their French fries as they attempt to finish their dinners. Rob's hyperactive mind matches his body. His thoughts chase one another at record speeds like drivers on the NASCAR circuit. They focus on the future, obsessing over minor things: *Did I double-check for bugs in that program? What if I can't get the second week in September off? If I go out with the guys tomorrow night, will Debbie give me the silent treatment?* His voice mails to friends are hard to understand; he talks so fast that they need to play his messages twice. Rob's body and mind are always wired for action, which makes it difficult for him to rest. He suffers from insomnia and wakes up frequently during the night. He wishes he could turn off his mind but says it's like a light switch, permanently set to the "on" position.

Rob came to his first private yoga therapy session reluctantly, sporting the belief that yoga was "for chicks only." He preferred activities such as weight training and running that felt to him like a physical workout. Yet just before I met him, Rob had an accident with his company car. His driver's license was suspended, and his insomnia worsened. Suddenly, he was more motivated to try yoga. Rob's therapeutic practice consisted of Sun Salutations, followed by the Anxiety-Balancing restorative sequence (chapter 8) and 1:2 Breathing (page 72). He emerged from his first session noticeably calmer, but still skeptical, and made a bet with me that the effects wouldn't last. I agreed to the bet on one condition: he had to do the breathwork at least once a day. To Rob's surprise, he liked 1:2 Breathing and practiced it three times daily. Restorative Yoga, on the other hand, was harder for Rob to commit to; it challenged his gym mind-set. Even so, he agreed to try it for six weeks to see if it would help. At the end of Restorative Yoga's "probationary period,"

Rob felt much more tranquil. He decided to do the practice for just ten to fifteen minutes daily after working out. Within two months, he was impressed enough with the results to commit to a regular practice. He recently even taught Face-Down Relaxation Pose from his restorative sequence to one of his stressed-out weight-room buddies.

Does the Anxious Body/Anxious Mind emotional type fit you? If it does (and your body is agitated and your mind is anxious, with racing thoughts), you share with Rob the straightforward type of body-mind anxiety. You are likely, during times of stress, to become anxious. You are less inclined, though it is still possible, to become depressed. You can find the practice that works best for your type, the Anxiety-Balancing Practice, in chapter 8. This practice brings calm to both the body and the mind. If parts of Rob's description fit you and parts did not, see whether one of the other types seems to better reflect the current state of your mind and body.

Emotional Type 2:
Depressed Body/Depressed Mind

The Depressed Body/Depressed Mind form of emotional imbalance means that you feel depression in both your both body and your mind. Linea came to me for help with her depression. From the moment we met, it was clear that she fit this emotional type to a T. Her shoulders and upper back rounded forward. She suffered from back pain and acknowledged that her core body (abdominal) muscles were weak. She slumped into the back of her chair for support, which shortened her midsection, and she appeared so exhausted that she could barely hold herself upright. Linea's marked listlessness was almost contagious; she yawned frequently and punctuated every few sentences with a gigantic sigh, saying, "I'm so tired, it's hard to keep going." When it came time to practice, Linea moved slowly and with great effort, as though she carried a hundred-pound weight on her back.

Linea's poor concentration and spotty memory interfered with her job performance as a paralegal. Despite her lovely smile and shy admission that she enjoyed yoga, Linea seemed so withdrawn at times that she nearly disappeared into herself. Her first yoga therapy session was punctuated by self-deprecating comments such as "I'm so out of shape right now" and "My hips are bad." She was slow to respond to my questions and laughed self-consciously when it took her so long to answer that she lost track of the original thread of conversation. Linea had tried several different antidepressants, but the medications she'd taken for the past two years were beginning to lose their effectiveness. Recently, Linea's outlook on life became even more negative and pessimistic: her daily mantra was "I'm such a loser; not even meds work for me." Linea wanted to begin private yoga therapy because she felt better after practicing yoga, but couldn't drag herself to classes often enough. Her sister and her best friend were worried, and urged Linea to see me before things got much worse.

Because Linea had a more straightforward depression that affected both her body and mind, she followed the Depression-Lifting Practice (chapter 9), which included back-bending poses to energize her body and 1:1 Breathing to keep her mind alert. After her second month of regular practice, her posture improved dramatically and she felt increased energy. Her thinking was less negative and more hopeful, and she felt motivated to practice yoga. Linea's improvement was slower than Rob's (depression can improve more gradually than anxiety, and her lethargy and sadness still waylaid her at times). However, after one year of weekly practice on her own plus one or two yoga therapy sessions per month, Linea felt as though she'd "re-entered the human race." She recently spoke to her psychiatrist, and with his approval and guidance, plans to taper off her antidepressant medication.

If Linea's physical and mental sluggishness sound familiar, you too may have the more straightforward type of depression. You are inclined, during times of stress, to become even more depressed and less apt, though it is still possible, to become anxious. The yoga practice most likely to work best for you is the Depression-Lifting Practice Linea followed, which helps increase energy in both the body and the mind.

Emotional Type 3:
Depressed Body/Anxious Mind

The next two types of emotional imbalance can be more difficult to identify because they involve mixtures of anxiety and depression. The difficulty centers on identifying which parts of us—body and/or mind—are depressed, and which are anxious. This is why check-ins are so important; they help us differentiate the body's symptoms from the mind's symptoms, so that we can treat them both effectively using yoga.

The first of the mixed emotional types, Depressed Body/Anxious Mind, is more common than the second. This first form of mixed emotional imbalance, which I call "Anxious Depression," means that you have physical symptoms of depression but mental signs of anxiety. Jen, one of my students, initially thought she was just depressed, as many people do who suffer from this type of emotional imbalance. Physically, her body resembled Linea's: her shoulders were rounded, and she often crossed her arms in front of her as though to protect her heart from injury. She had difficulty breathing, and typically inhaled and exhaled through her mouth slowly and shallowly. Jen's movements were also listless; in yoga class, her energy burned out quickly, and she spent a lot of time resting in Child's Pose or excusing herself to go to the bathroom. "I feel like a truck ran over me," she often said.

Despite her physical lethargy, Jen experienced a good deal of mental anxiety. With the slightest provocation, her mind raced. She often worried about what people thought of her. She was afraid of not keeping up at her job, and pressured herself to work harder. She had performance anxiety in yoga class as well; anytime I asked her to demonstrate something, she would freeze and say, "I can't remember what I'm supposed to do!" Jen struggled with medication: although it improved her physical lethargy, it intensified her mental agitation. Her doctor prescribed Xanax to take the edge off her anxiety, but Jen didn't like the way it made her feel.

Jen displayed the physical expression of depression, but the mental pattern of anxiety. She used the first sequence in chapter 10, which provided back-bending restorative postures to bring more energy to her body and reverse Closed Heart Syndrome (see page 213). The practice also included 1:2 Breathing to calm her mind. Because Jen didn't do anything halfway, she practiced this sequence every day. The results were amazing: in only six weeks, Jen's mind was calmer. She no longer needed Xanax during the day and used it only once or twice to help her sleep. She had greater physical energy and more motivation for tasks she usually avoided. She was able to lower her dosage of antidepressants, yet still felt their benefits.

If your body is sluggish and low in energy like Linea's, but your mind is more agitated like Rob's or Jen's, you may have "Anxious Depression." You are likely, during times of stress, to become more physically depleted, yet more mentally agitated. Furthermore, most treatments (whether medication or yoga) that are designed to increase your energy can also awaken a dormant mental anxiety. The suggested yoga practice for you is for Depressed Body/Anxious Mind, the first practice in chapter 10. The restorative poses in this practice build energy in the body, while the breathwork ratio of 1:2 keeps the mind balanced and calm.

Emotional Type 4:
Anxious Body/Depressed Mind

The Anxious Body/Depressed Mind type of emotional imbalance involves the physical symptoms of anxiety but the mental characterdistics of depression. Of the four types, this is the rarest. Luis, a young client from my psychotherapy practice, had this type of emotional imbalance, which you can think of as "Depressed Anxiety." His body was so full of energy that he found it hard to calm down. Luis often worked out twice a day and lifted weights in the evening, despite the fact that his muscles, particularly his neck, were already contracted with pain and stiffness. Luis preferred to do everything fast. He literally ran wherever he went, and was often impatient with friends and family who lived their lives at a more natural pace. When he was forced to sit still, like in meetings at the graphic design firm where he worked, his physical agitation became more pronounced. To the great annoyance of his colleagues,

Luis would click his retractable pen on and off, or fold and twist pieces of paper into different shapes.

In contrast to the frenetic pace of his body, Luis's mind felt immersed in quicksand. He had trouble generating ideas for projects or would simply forget them from one moment to the next. His thoughts came slowly, and his speech was so delayed that his friends and family typically finished his sentences. Sometimes he seemed anxious or even hyperactive, and other times completely depressed and lethargic. His parents were exasperated with Luis and didn't know how to help him.

Because Luis's body had physical manifestations of anxiety but his mental state was more characteristic of depression, he benefited from the forward-bending Restorative Yoga sequence with 1:1 Breathing (page 213), the second sequence in chapter 10. Luis immediately took to the forward-bending restorative poses, which slowed his body down. He practiced 1:1 Breathing, and at first found inhaling much harder than exhaling. It took him two months, but he eventually learned to balance his inhale and exhale. To Luis, the equal inhale and exhale felt energizing, and helped him stay focused and alert.

If your body matches Luis's and Rob's in agitation, but your mind is sluggish like Linea's, you may have "Depressed Anxiety." During times of stress, your body is liable to grow even more agitated, while your mind may become slower and less alert. Treatments designed primarily to calm your physical agitation can slow your thinking too much. The yoga practice that will likely work best for you is the one Luis practiced, for Anxious Body/Depressed Mind. The restorative poses in this sequence help calm and ground the body, while the breathwork ratio of 1:1 keeps the mind more alert.

Choosing Your Breathwork and Restorative Yoga Sequence

Each time you get ready to practice, take a few moments in a quiet space to tune in to your body and mind. If necessary, review the four types of emotional imbalance in this chapter so you can tailor your practice to how you're feeling at the moment. Whether you've chosen the Anxiety-Balancing, Depression-Lifting, or Balancing Mixed Anxiety and Depression practices, do a check-in during and after each pose. This will help you maintain awareness of how the breathwork and restorative postures affect your body and your mind, and also enable you to fine-tune your sequence right in the middle of your practice. Your body, your mind, and your awareness will also help you notice if you've shifted from your "normal" emotional imbalance type and, either temporarily or for a longer period of time, moved into another. It's natural to fluctuate between types; check in with yourself regularly to note any fluctuations and adjust your practice accordingly.

Checking in also helps you identify physical discomfort, which can turn on your sympathetic (emergency response) system. If your body becomes uncomfortable during a pose, consider the possible sources of your discomfort. It could be physical, either because you're not supporting yourself fully, or because the pose itself is not right for you. Your discomfort could also be emotional, because strong emotions have surfaced during the practice. When you first feel physical discomfort in any part of your body, direct your breath to that part for one to two minutes, and see if your breath can relax it. If the discomfort persists longer than a couple of minutes, try the following:

1. Add more support to the pose.
2. If support doesn't provide relief, change your breath ratio.
3. If neither of these adjustments works, move on to the next pose in the sequence.
4. If nothing you've tried has helped, transition to a neutral restorative pose.

Let's use the forward-bending (face-down) poses as an example. When you are in Child's Pose or Reclining Twist, you may experience discomfort. First, question whether your discomfort is physical or emotional. If it's physical, let's go through the four steps together:

1. Does your breathing feel constricted? If so, you may need more propping for your shoulders. Try making "shoulder

pads" to open your chest a little, by placing folded hand towels under each shoulder for support (see instructions, page 233, on propping Child's Pose).

2. If adding more support doesn't work, make sure you're breathing in the right ratio (a longer exhale or 1:2 Breathing for an overactive mind or 1:1 Breathing for a sluggish mind). If need be, change your breath ratio.

3. If you can't get comfortable in a forward-bending pose no matter what support and breathing you've tried, give yourself permission to move on to the next pose in the sequence.

4. If you continue to feel discomfort in the forward-bending poses, transition to a neutral pose (where you are neither forward bending nor opening your heart too much), such as Side-Lying Pose or Legs-up-the-Wall Pose. As a final option, you can always consider whether your body might have depression while your mind has anxiety. If you think this might be the case, try the back-bending restorative sequence and use 1:2 Breathing to keep your mind calm.

If your discomfort is not physical but emotional, the best thing you can do is focus on your inhale and exhale. Breathe through your emotions. Allow them to be present without needing to become involved in them. If possible, release them a little bit with each exhale. (For additional guidance with this, see the Going with the Flow of Emotions exercise [page 128] and also the suggestions in chapter 7 [pages 151–54] for dealing with the emotional effects of these practices.) These recommendations for addressing discomfort also apply to the back-bending Restorative Yoga poses (see page 225 for more details).

Each sequence of postures offers recommended poses. You'll naturally be drawn to some poses more than others, so it's fine to deviate from these sequences. Each sequence also offers recommended timings that indicate how long to remain in that pose. You'll notice that a wide range of time is given in each pose so that you have the freedom to relax deeply or change poses. This also helps your body access its wisdom. As long as you're comfort-

able, if you feel that a certain pose is powerful or deeply relaxing—
in other words, if it "speaks" to you—feel free to stay in it for the
maximum length of time recommended (in some cases, up to one
hour). You can even choose to do only one pose throughout your
practice, if that feels best. Do make sure, however, that you don't
exceed the outer limit of timings for that pose and that you
don't experience any discomfort. Conversely, you can also skip a
pose that your body doesn't like (even if you're initially comfortable in it), and move on to another pose in the sequence. Remember
to let your body make the decision whether to remain or move on,
rather than feeling pressured to do the practice exactly as it's written. The more awareness you build in your mind and body, and the
more you inhabit your body, the better able you'll be to discern and
honor what works best for you.

Using Your Breath to Refine the Practice

Breath has a rapid effect on the nervous system, and thus also on
your mind. In the four practices that follow, in chapters 8–10, you
can use your breath as a minute-by-minute intervention to regulate,
soothe, or energize your thoughts. If your mind is anxious and your
thoughts are racing, use a longer exhale or 1:2 Breathing (see page
72) to calm them. If your mind remains active, you can increase the
ratio to 1:3 or more, allowing your exhale to be at least three times
as long as your inhale. On the other hand if your mind is slow and
your thoughts are sluggish, try 1:1 Breathing (see page 48), in which
your inhale and exhale are equal. This will keep your mind energized
and calm at the same time. (In case you are wondering why you can't
inhale longer than you exhale to increase mental energy, breathing
in a way that emphasizes the inhale too much is similar to hyperventilation and can create or exacerbate anxiety.)

If at first you find the breathing practices difficult, don't worry.
When you've experienced anxiety or high stress for a long time,
lengthening your exhale may initially be challenging. Turn to the
Getting to Know Your Breath exercise (page 28) and simply breathe
in and out through your nose. In time, you can progress to 1:1
Breathing, making your inhale and exhale equal in length. When

you are comfortable with an equal inhale-to-exhale ratio, you can experiment by lengthening your exhale. Maintain a longer exhale until it feels comfortable. Eventually, your exhale will be twice as long as your inhale. It may take several sessions (or weeks or even months) to get used to your target breath ratio. If so, that's normal. Patience is important in learning to regulate your breath. Remember that you've lived with your old (and likely shallow) breathing pattern for many years. It may take a little time and patient effort to change it.

Growing New Patterns

In the beginning, practicing a new behavior (such as deeper breathing, relaxation, or being present in your body) takes determination. The new behavior is weaker than the old, habitual one; it hasn't yet become a pattern in its own right. During this gestational period, the fledgling behavior is vulnerable. It requires energy, focus, and dedication to grow stronger. As your practice matures, you may notice subtle signs of discomfort that invite you to support yourself differently or alter your sequence to fit your mood. Pay attention to these signs. Your emotional baseline may also change from day to day. Listen to these changes. Doing so will help you adjust your practice and thereby increase its effectiveness. Don't force yourself to fit the practices in this book; give yourself permission to let the practices fit *you.*

7

The Heart of the Practice

ONCE YOU IDENTIFY YOUR EMOTIONAL TYPE, THEN THE outer structure (the *form*) of your practice falls into place. In therapeutic yoga we honor the form, yet also look beyond it. We focus on the inner nature (the *essence*) of the practice. As you might expect, people often find the form, the breathing exercises and restorative poses, relatively simple. They discover that the essence, what happens when we practice, is more challenging. Why does the essence of the practice even matter in shifting anxiety and depression? In this chapter, we'll find out. We'll also delve into some of the common challenges that can arise in the practice, and explore ways of meeting them.

As with most contemplative practices, yoga doesn't erase difficulty; it illuminates it. When the body stays in one place, our baggage comes flying out of storage. This happens almost before we begin: our expectations for the practice, and for ourselves, emerge. We get to take them out, dust them off, and determine whether we still have use for them. Zoe, a student in one of my Restorative Yoga weekend workshops, came face-to-face with one of her major issues early on. At first, she sought a state of *perfect relaxation*. She mentally evaluated each aspect of the poses, from the quality of her props (the blankets weren't smooth enough) to the alignment of her body (her tighter left hip made the poses "crooked"). The room wasn't warm enough or dark enough for her to relax deeply. All her attention went to the props, and the excess mental activity pushed her nervous system into overdrive. It took Zoe two months of circling around the practice to realize that her perfectionism on the mat reflected the way she approached her life off the mat. Her exceedingly high performance standards prevented her from trying new things—or things she couldn't immediately master. All this helped her avoid any feelings of anger, sadness, or vulnerability. With time and encouragement, Zoe learned not to fixate on the outer details. Gradually, she allowed herself to "drop into" the poses and experience her emotions. When she did, she found Restorative Yoga to be a container for feeling and releasing difficult emotions more fluidly than she'd thought possible.

Setting the Stage for Practice

Every restorative class I teach begins with an invitation to "make the practice your own." I let people know that they can practice one pose for the entire class, choose a couple they like, or try every pose in the sequence. Yet practitioners still regularly ask me, "What am I supposed to be doing here?" or "What should this pose look like?" The elusive idea of doing the "right thing" and being a good student can rear its head even in a restorative practice. But in Restorative Yoga, more so than any other practice, you have permission to leave the *shoulds* and the *supposed tos* behind. Although the sequences in part 2 include recommended timings, step-by-step instructions, and alignment suggestions, you're not meant simply to follow a script. Instead, you're asked to evolve the self-awareness that you started to build in part 1, and follow your body's lead. Yet how, exactly, do you do this?

First of all, in an active yoga practice you might be tempted to measure your performance through flexibility, strength, or alignment. A restorative practice, however, is internal. There's no easy way to gauge how well you do, so you can let go of the need to be a good student. Your practice can be a setting for experimentation, like a scientist's laboratory. The experimentation doesn't need to progress in an orderly way; it can be spontaneous and creative. This nicely contrasts a common expectation you might encounter in your life outside the practice: that you follow directions and not experience anything out of the ordinary. Allow your practice to become a refuge for self-study, for research on yourself. Try out different breathwork ratios and restorative postures, and observe how your mind and body receive them. This opens you up to chance encounters with hidden parts of yourself. You don't need to do anything to evoke these hidden parts; they'll emerge on their own. Some may be delightful, and others painful. You may be tempted to welcome certain parts, such as the intuitive, assertive, or creative parts, and stuff others back in the closet. The thing is, the energy it takes to suppress the "bad" stuff will also stifle the good. Opening up to the good, the bad, and the neutral will help you develop equanimity to all of your emotional experiences.

When the Practice Is Difficult

Most of us don't travel lightly through life. We may create the illusion that we do by trying to outrun our difficulties. We may attempt to "lose" our baggage by flying, as fast as we can, from one place to the next. Yet as soon as we land at our next destination, there's our baggage: circling on the carousel, waiting for us to pick it up. We need to claim it so that it's not always there, one step ahead, waiting for us. We need to experience it fully before we can let it go.

You may be surprised when issues you thought you'd worked through in therapy or self-study suddenly re-emerge in a restorative practice. You may wonder, "Haven't I dealt with this already?" Christopher, a regular in Restorative Yoga class, had been in therapy for over twelve years, learning to manage his negative thinking and low self-esteem. Through therapy he'd become more positive and confident. Still, as happens for most of us, a residue of depression remained in his body and mind. For the first several months of restorative practice, Christopher struggled with his hopeless outlook: he feared that the practice would never help and that he was "bad at it anyway." He doubted his ability to get himself into the poses correctly. When he did manage to do them, he insisted he was "practically senile" and wouldn't remember how to re-create the support and alignment he'd just managed to generate. Although

Christopher's self-esteem had improved in therapy, the practice un-covered another layer that his body still needed to process.

In Restorative Yoga, a wide range of issues can come up. A harsh inner critic can catalog your faults. A catastrophic mind-set can accelerate your nervous system. Old feelings about your body can percolate up to the surface. Strange aches and pains can come and go. You may even encounter experiences that have never been triggered before. If these things happen, embrace them; they are a living, breathing part of your practice.

People often ask me why difficult thoughts and feelings come up during, of all settings, Restorative Yoga. The answer is that when you relax your body and quiet your mind, you can begin to *viscerally* process and let go of stored emotions. If you've never had this happen before, you may feel a little alarmed, or wonder if the prac-tice is making you worse. Don't be concerned; most of the time, the surfacing of emotion is actually a sign that the practice is doing what it's meant to. Remember that you don't need to talk about, think about, or even understand what comes up in your practice in order to let it go. Instead, you can simply *allow*. Allow any thoughts, emotions, or experiences to come and go at their own pace.

Through yoga, you can bring compassionate, neutral observation to your issues. You can stay sympathetic instead of judgmental, neutral rather than biased. What helps you do this? The basics of the practice: breath and relaxation, which are tools you've already encountered. When you focus on your breath and relax your body, you open more to direct experience. Here, you are not good, not bad. You simply *are*.

When challenges come up in your practice, let your breath an-chor you. In my Restorative Yoga classes, we use a "trick" that helps: Imagine that challenging thoughts and feelings are like thun-derclouds in the sky. Focus on your breath. Become aware of each part of your inhale from beginning to end. No matter what comes up, continue to focus on the breath. Use your exhale to "blow" these thunderclouds away. When you're stirred up, you can use 1:2 Breathing (or 1:1 Breathing, if the former is harder) to help difficult emotions move through you. This can help you to acknowledge and observe your emotions without getting caught up in them. In time, you can choose to do the same with positive experiences as well. Why might you want to do this? Both positive and negative experiences are temporary, and holding on makes them more permanent. When you practice observing and letting go of all experiences—positive, negative, or neutral—you tune in to the essential transience of anxiety and depression.

For some people, these techniques might not be enough to tolerate a direct experience of the mind, body, and emotions. This was the case for Kara, a Vinyasa and Restorative Yoga practitioner. Kara oscillated between intense physical and mental agitation, and intense physical and mental lethargy. In an active, moving yoga practice, she felt relatively safe. In Restorative Yoga, however, she couldn't tolerate the intense pressure-cooker feelings that came up when her body was still. She'd grow irritable and restless, and each practice would give rise to a struggle of epic proportions. Understandably, Kara felt miserable when she practiced. I advised her to back off a little and stay in a restorative posture for only five minutes at a time, or as long as she could handle. When she reached her maximum tolerance level, she could transition into a new pose. If she needed to take a break entirely, I encouraged her to get water or use the bathroom while continuing to breathe mindfully and stay as relaxed as possible. Kara felt bad about not being able to "do it right." Yet as I told her, the restorative practice is not an "equanimity contest." She could benefit just as much from shorter periods in each pose. With encouragement, Kara gave herself permission to practice shorter sequences and to get up and move around when necessary. The shorter intervals of practice instilled a sense of safety and calm. She began to observe her frustration and self-imposed pressure to perform. The more she observed her experiences without judgment, the more they softened. Slowly, her periods of anxiety grew less intense. Her episodes of depression began to lift. She approached the practice in a looser, less performance-oriented way. Although within six months, Kara was able to practice for forty-five minutes without needing a break, she found that length of practice became less important.

What matters every bit as much as a "good practice" is a practice that doesn't work as well as you'd like. How do you treat yourself when you don't "perform" well? How do you address the parts of the practice that don't seem to go smoothly? How do you relate to yourself when you sneak only a five-minute restorative pose into a frenetic day or when you worry throughout an entire practice? Do you listen to the instincts that suggest you stay in Reclining Twist for longer than you'd planned? And if you fall asleep during the practice for the tenth time in a row, how do you handle that? These moments (when you are restless, when challenging feelings come up, or when you fall asleep, for example) are encounters with the unexpected. They may be the most important points in your journey. In these moments, your gentle self-observation and the friendly witnessing of your own experience matter most. Your non-judgment and self-compassion help you develop mental flexibility and open-mindedness. They challenge the performance-oriented, closed-minded neural networks of anxiety and depression.

When the Practice Is Easy and Life Is Difficult

Everywhere we look, it seems, we're flooded with images of instant Zen: a tanned, relaxed woman dressed in white sits effortlessly in lotus position, thumbs and index fingers touching in yoga mudra. A shirtless, muscular-backed guy rests soulfully in Child's Pose. An attractive young couple strolls hand in hand along a beach as the sun sets. These glossy images can transmit the notion that when we practice yoga, our lives will be just as idyllic.

Tracy, a student of mine, once remarked mournfully that while her practice on the mat made her feel really "blissed-out," the rest of her life was a problem. After yoga class, Tracy felt open to a vast array of possibilities. She could live a more meaningful, connected life (she imagined a wide network of friends and extended family). She could use her talents as an artist and healer to help others (she visualized working with orphans in Haiti). She could be a better, more responsive daughter to her parents (she vowed to return their calls more often). She could be more understanding with Jason, her husband (she imagined not castigating him for every tiny character flaw). For a brief period, life appeared to be wonderful. . . . Then class would end and she'd go home. Jason would do something to set her off: dinner wouldn't be ready or he'd leave his underwear on the bathroom floor. Within minutes of her "incredible" yoga class, she and her husband would lock horns. "Doesn't he get it?" she asked me. "I just want to preserve the bliss for a few hours— I'll even take fifteen minutes! But each time I come home, he gets on my nerves!" She couldn't understand why life wasn't more like yoga. A couple of years later, Tracy brought Jason to class. "Great class," he said on his way out. "But I've gotta tell you—at first I really resented yoga. I couldn't figure out why, every Tuesday night after class, Tracy was such a raving lunatic. I mean, yoga's supposed to make people mellower, right?"

Sometimes our practice can seem like the easy part. It can provide a sanctuary from our problems, a newfound equilibrium, and a brief sense of insulation from our own or others' toxic emotions. We can feel momentarily protected from the issues that are often thrown at us when we engage deeply with others and with life. We may not want to test this fragile equilibrium out in the world. But among all the yoga teachers I have studied alongside, learned from, and befriended, one common thread of philosophical discussion often comes up: Do we practice (yoga or meditation) for our own enlightenment? Or is our practice meant to be taken off the mountaintop or mat and into the world? In my opinion, we don't balance the nervous system, regulate the breath, tune in to direct experience, and quiet the mind to be emotionally balanced in isolation. We do so to connect better with ourselves, others, and the world. But this process of connection begins with the body.

Letting Your Body Run the Show

Every Thursday evening for the past seven years or so, I've taught a Restorative Yoga class. This class functions as a laboratory, not only for my students' learning but my own. We gain knowledge about the relationship between mind and body, about the therapeutic nature of the practice, and about what helps relieve mental and emotional suffering the most. Based on my observations, I've made changes: I've fine-tuned the sequence of postures for anxiety, depression, and insomnia. I've shifted the way postures are propped.

Yet the most significant changes have been in relation to the psychology and not the physiology of the practice.

Many practitioners are challenged at two key points in the class. The first comes right at the beginning: As the class starts, I ask everyone to come to their mats. I emphasize that the most significant part of the class, checking in, occurs right here and now, and that it may be one of the hardest parts. I start a simple, two-minute check-in. I ask them to close their eyes, tune in to their bodies, and assess their energy level. They are asked to pick one of the following: overenergized, totally tired, or somewhere in the middle. This helps set the stage for the shape of restorative postures (grounding or heart-opening) they will try. But despite my invitations to investigate what's going on inside, usually several people get up to search for props. And even though I remind them that the class is not about me but about them, some keep their gaze trained on me. Like baby birds, eyes wide open, they scan me as if I could drop all the remedies for life's ailments into their beaks. It is, indeed, so hard to go inward.

The second key juncture in the restorative practice has also taught me how hard it is for us to listen to and honor our body's needs. For example, you have several opportunities either to stay where you are or to change positions and move into a different pose. For the first several years of teaching, at these junctures I'd say something like, "And now you can either stay as you are or begin to transition up to sitting for 'X' Pose." Nearly everyone (except advanced practitioners) dutifully transitioned out of the pose and into the next. They did this even when they appeared to be deeply relaxed, comfortable, and largely content before moving. Sometimes they'd say to me afterward, "I really loved Relaxation Pose. I could've stayed there for the whole class!" When I'd tell them that they could in fact do that, they'd sort of shrug, smile, and thank me for the class. I wondered why, even when given permission to stay, did people move out of positions they loved and that clearly worked wonders for them? The answer seems to lie in the habit of doing what we're told, of seeking approval even in the subtlest of ways. I wondered if somehow, the way I'd worded the instrsuctions caused people to want to do what they thought I wanted.

I began to tell the class up front that following the body's lead would enhance their practice. Each time I offered a new pose, I instructed them to check in briefly. If their body wanted to change positions, they could let their body make that choice. If it felt as though they were "dropping" deeper into the practice and their body wanted to stay, they could stay. Suddenly, I witnessed a dramatic shift: most people opted to stay. Since that simple change in instruction, the vast majority of our practitioners consistently choose only one to three poses throughout their practice instead of a possible five to six. The assistants have remarked on how deeply relaxed people seem to be.

Often, the mind tells the body what to do. The mind's need to override the body's wisdom and comfort can interfere with the benefits of our yoga practice. At a recent weekend workshop, I saw this drive to be a good student in action. I advised the participants that they might experience physical discomfort in a restorative posture, and if this were to occur, they should breathe through it and see if the breath could bring some ease—but to do so for no more than a couple of minutes. After the first restorative practice, however, several participants admitted that they'd experienced an increase in anxiety. When we explored this further, they said that it was due to prolonged discomfort in one of the poses. And yet, they remained in the pose because it felt like something they "should do." Together, we connected this incident to the helplessness that can cause people with anxiety and depression to tolerate physically and emotionally painful situations without attempting to adjust them. They all expressed a *mental understanding* of this, and I invited them to come out of a pose the next time they felt a discomfort that the breath could not assuage. Later that afternoon, several people again reported an increase in mental anxiety. Curious, I asked how many of these had also experienced *physical* discomfort, and was surprised to see three quarters of the class raise their hands. Jokingly, I asked how many of those who'd just raised their hands had also remained in a state of discomfort earlier in the day. Nearly half had done so. They shared an embarrassed chuckle before one person explained that despite my permission to come out, she'd still felt that she "should" stay. We acknowledged as a group how challenging it is to change the belief that we should submit to painful situations. We can carry this pattern of thinking even when we don't need to, and when we know that discomfort is counterproductive for our growth.

When we allow the mind to step aside, the body's innate knowledge and authority can emerge. It's not that the mind creates a "bad" practice—it's that the body designs a practice with more organic integrity. So when you practice, allow your body's comfort to dictate when, or whether, it wants to move to a new pose. Let your body lead, and you'll be surprised by what happens.

The Journey versus the Destination

Modern culture tends to emphasize the *outcome* of what we do rather than the *process*. Like a child on a long car ride, you can feel the persistent question "Are we there yet?" bursting inside. In the face of anxiety or depression, you may work hard to make things better. You might read books, exercise more regularly, find the right support group, talk to a therapist, take medication, or seek natural ways to heal. You may also try to talk yourself out of a place of anxiety or depression. Often, these *try hard* methods don't turn out as planned. What's more, "working on" yourself mirrors the high expectations and relentless internal pressure of anxiety and depression, even if you don't intend it to.

Not long ago, one of my students came up after class to lodge a complaint. Lyle had practiced Restorative Yoga for about three months. He felt great after class, he told me: totally calm and with a renewed sense of connection. He felt more confident in himself, both professionally and personally. His depression had really improved. Yet why, as soon as he sat down in front of his boss, did all the assertive things he'd planned to say fly out of his mind? What's the benefit of regular practice, he asked, if it doesn't change our behavior? As I told Lyle, if you expect to "get it" right away, to feel emotionally balanced after only a few tries, you could be setting yourself up for disappointment.

In part 1, you learned five ways to transform your emotional patterns: calming the nervous system, regulating the breath, connecting with direct experience, quieting the mind, and changing the narratives (the filter) that reflect your self-concept and world view. If you've suffered from anxiety or depression for a long time, this may be hard to believe, but the greatest value of these healing methods lies not in their results. Instead, the value can be found in the carefree way you approach the journey and in the adventures and detours that come along the way. Yet whether we're looking for creative inspiration, emotional balance, or spiritual fulfillment, the journey itself, the process, is the most important and healing part.

Finding inspiration doesn't come just from intentions and deliberate work. Imagine for a moment that you're a scientist. Your research focuses on finding the cure for a rare kind of brain cancer. Of course, people have expectations of you—you have expectations of yourself. For some people, your research is a life-and-death matter. To find the cure for this disease, you might think you should work harder, faster, better. Many of the great discoveries in science, medicine, art, music, teaching, and personal and creative endeavors (such as yoga) can be accidental. They often happen when the mind and body play and explore.

For this exploration we have to become more relaxed about making mistakes, a prospect that can ignite anxiety even in the most mature among us. Some of the key insights that have shaped my personal practice and teaching have caught me by surprise. I've expected them to show up as a reward for hard work. I've thought they would come while I was chained to my desk for the twelfth straight hour. I've imagined they'd hit me in the midst of reading my fourteenth book on a topic that I "should" research. I may have spent hours poring over something with little inspiration. Doubtless, the many hours of preparation have made a contribution. Nonetheless, there it is: inspiration, when my mind and body are at play, and not immersed in hard work or in the need to get things *right*. The most valuable insights tend to arrive when I'm practicing on my mat, deep in meditation, swimming at my local pond, playing with children, or preparing a meal. Try to play a bit in your pratice, and see where it takes you.

Great Expectations

Recently, a friend announced she was quitting a pottery class she'd raved about for the last year. I asked why, slightly dismayed (I'd been the beneficiary of two very nice oversized saffron-colored latte mugs). Seeing my surprise, she explained: "I'm terrible at it. I'll never be as good as I want to be, so why keep going?" I felt sad for her. Yet I've reflected on and even felt this tendency many times. It's in our childhood nature to play, to immerse ourselves in direct experience. But our adult nature wants to be good at things. This can lead us to value being good over simply *being*.

In each Restorative Yoga class I teach, people ask, "What should I be feeling?" or "Is this how the pose is supposed to look?" They can immobilize themselves with worry that if they don't execute a pose perfectly or feel what they're supposed to feel, they'll fail. It's ironic: searching for the perfect relaxation pose or practice actually undermines relaxation. To relax, you need to let go of perfection. The drive toward perfection and achievement is universal; we see it everywhere. It's also an inherent part of the "great expectations" of anxiety and depression. Furthermore, this drive is the opposite of what we need. It precludes relaxation. It blocks self-compassion. It blinds awareness. And relaxation, self-compassion, and awareness are key ingredients in emotional balance.

Like others, you may play the comparison game, and evaluate yourself in relation to something or someone else. The comparison game can cause you to label yourself as "good" or "bad." Yet labeling makes it nearly impossible to learn about yourself through trial and error, through exploration. Think for a moment of exercising. You can fall into the expectation that if you exercise once or twice, you should be in good shape or if you practice something a few times, you should be able to master it. You can then get upset if you have a bad practice. Yet, in yoga, there's no such thing as a "good" or "bad" practice. Practice simply means to put something into action and do it frequently. It also means to learn by repetition.

This book's use of the word *practice* is not accidental; the concept of practice is an inherent part of yoga philosophy. Doing the exercises in this book—practicing them—is a way to engage not just with the mind but with the body, as often as possible, even on a daily basis. It took decades of practice to get us to our present emotional state, to work our mental, neural, and physical muscles into patterns of anxiety or depression. Why would we expect only one or two sessions of yoga to undo those effects?

For the purpose of this book, it's helpful to think of the exercises and practices as just that: a chance to unlearn anxiety and depression and relearn equanimity and balance. You do this through the repetition of actions in a practice, but also by remaining open to whatever you can discover about yourself.

Restorative Yoga doesn't require (externally, at least) much active doing. So it challenges the part of us that needs to be productive every minute of every day. We often try to co-opt yoga as a vehicle for an extreme makeover, doggedly attempting to make ourselves better, stronger, more flexible, calmer, as though there were something deeply wrong with us. But yoga emphasizes nonstriving. All of yoga's philosophical texts encourage us to practice with dedication and intensity, but also without an agenda. In other words, forget self-improvement. Try practicing self-compassion instead.

Let go of the idea that you can either do well at the practice or fail at it. If the idea of being good or bad at yoga stubbornly persists, you can just choose to acknowledge it as you breathe in, and release any fantasies of being good or fears of failing as you breathe out. In working toward emotional balance, try to be as childlike as you can. Let go of the need to turn your practice into a good performance. Instead, just see where it takes you.

Support and Self-Care

To prop means to "support" or "sustain." In the practice of yoga, a prop is anything you use to support or sustain you. In Western Yoga, props are often something you "lean on," a crutch until you can do the pose "without help." In Restorative Yoga, props such as bolsters or blankets are an essential part of the practice. They provide you the support you need to hold poses for longer periods of time. They minimize muscular contraction. They help quiet your blood pressure, heart rate, and brain function, and they promote the relaxation response of your rest-and-digest system. On a concrete level, they're fairly simple to use. On a symbolic level, it's another story.

In my active Vinyasa classes, I often encounter students who resist props: "I don't need that," they say. "I'm flexible—I can do the pose without it!" Sometimes, it's hard to accept support. Props can contradict the work ethic that may have formed the backdrop of your upbringing. Or perhaps you're used to comfort and support, but on a more superficial level. You may have learned to indulge in expensive cars, clothes, or cosmetic maintenance rituals while denying yourself true self-care.

Yvette, a young woman who usually practiced the depression-lifting sequence, took my weekly Restorative Yoga classes for over five years and my Vinyasa classes for over seven. She was no stranger, then, to the concept of self-care. Yet many times, moving among the practitioners, I'd find that she would forgo support under her head, even though her neck hyperextended. And sometimes, she would practice a posture that required a blanket between the shins, such as Reclining Twist, without using a blanket—thus compressing her pelvis. I'd stop to point this out, and she'd laugh sheepishly and say that she was "too lazy" to use the necessary blanket or towel and didn't want to bother the class assistants. Yvette knew well the significance of propping for relaxation and calm. She wasn't lazy. She just had a habit (samskara) of sacrificing physical comfort in order to avoid the emotional discomfort of receiving.

Props support you. They help you nourish yourself. Here's the challenging part: if you have learned in life to pull yourself up by your bootstraps, swallow discomfort, or avoid asking for help, the idea of accepting "support" or "sustenance" can be foreign and unsettling. Recently, after two restorative classes, a woman with fibromyalgia wrote to me about her experience. "Why do we resist comfort and self-care?" she asked. "We often think being strong means we can't be vulnerable. But being vulnerable opens the door to health and healing when we need it. It helps the unconscious learn that we aren't alone. There's help that makes us stronger—no matter the poor parenting, the demands from family, the things that drain us. Being comforted, supported, and not constantly pushing actually makes us stronger." The use of props can raise certain questions: What do support and sustenance mean to you? How would it feel to allow someone or something to support you? What would it be like if you consistently nurtured yourself?

Physically, Restorative Yoga is easy. Emotionally, it's challenging because deep down, you may find comfort and support to be unnerving. Restorative Yoga asks that you commit to the lost art of self-care. If you're ambivalent about this, Restorative Yoga brings this ambivalence right to the forefront of your awareness. You may wonder, *Have I done enough today to justify relaxing? Have I taken care of everyone else before doing this for myself? Is it OK to get my needs met?* Comfort and self-care are essential to truly supporting your emotional well-being, so in your practice, please use the props and add the support your body asks for.

And now, on to the practice.

~8

Anxiety-Balancing Practice
Calming Your Body and Mind

ANXIETY-BALANCING PRACTICE IS DESIGNED FOR THOSE with Anxious Body/Anxious Mind, and those with Anxious Body/ Depressed Mind. It features forward-bending (face-down) restorative poses to ground, calm, and soothe your body. If you have an anxious mind, you will use 1:2 breathing (see page 72) to calm your mind and nervous system. But if your mind is already balanced or slow, you will use 1:1 Breathing (see page 48) to keep your mind calm, yet also alert.

Before beginning this practice, do a check-in to get your mental and physical baselines (see page 50 for more information) so you can measure any changes that occur as a result of the practice. Also include a mini-check-in between each pose, to help you develop a sense of how the pose you've just done has worked for you. Always feel free to remain in a pose for the maximum time recommended, or to practice only one or two poses, if that feels best to your body. Trust your body's wisdom to tell you what feels comfortable. In contrast to active yoga classes, which have a goal of stretching and outer work, Restorative Yoga emphasizes relaxation and inner work. Relaxation is important in changing your emotional patterns. Awareness of your direct experience, especially the ability to distinguish comfort from discomfort), will help you deepen relaxation, and balance your body and mind.

There is also an online audio version of this sequence, which gives you a guide for your practice (see page 8 for more details). Tracks 1–11 will talk you through getting into, and modifying, each pose and give you suggestions on how to direct your breath and awareness while you're there.

Anxiety-Balancing Posture Sequence

TRACKS 1–11

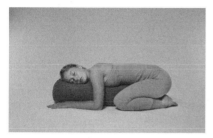

1. Child's Pose

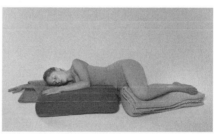

2. Reclining Twist

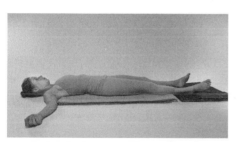

3. Inversion Pose

4. Side-Lying Pose

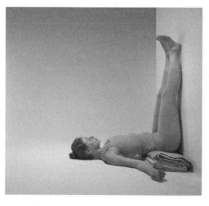

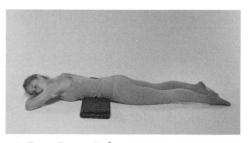

6. Face-Down Relaxation Pose

5. Legs-up-the-Wall Pose

⌒ CHILD'S POSE

Time: 5–10 *minutes*

TRACKS 2–3

PROPS

- 1 round bolster (or alternative; see page 228)
- 1–2 blankets
- 1 hand towel, folded lengthwise
- 1 eye pillow

A QUICK WORD ABOUT THIS POSE

Child's Pose is grounding, and can give you a sense of being enveloped in calm. Yet achieving comfort in this pose can take longer than you may have anticipated. If you use the props, you will be rewarded with increased comfort. I'll walk you through how to support yourself best in each pose. If this is your first time practicing, you may find it helpful to read the "Guidelines for Additional Support" section in order to better anticipate the potential areas of concern.

Remember that physical comfort is important. If you've tried the modifications and added extra support, and still feel discomfort in Child's Pose, you can leave it out of your sequence. You can begin your practice with Reclining Twist (page 170) instead.

INSTRUCTIONS

1. Place your bolster in the middle of your mat, lengthwise.

2. Kneel down just behind your bolster, so that you're facing it. Draw your knees a little wider than hips' width apart, and sit back on your heels.

3. Take a moment to check in with your body. You might be able to tell just by kneeling here whether you have any discomfort. Potential places for discomfort in this pose are the feet, knees, and hips. If you do feel discomfort, proceed to the "Guidelines for Additional Support" section below for help in supporting your body.

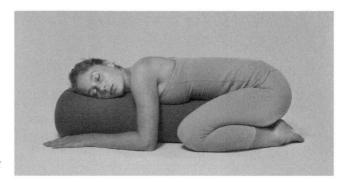

fig. 8.1

4. If you don't have any discomfort, lie down over the bolster. Rest your forearms on the mat with your elbows approximately under the shoulders, or wherever they feel most comfortable (fig. 8.1).

5. Take a moment to ensure that your hips and your head are fairly level, which means that you have sufficient bolster (or blanket) height, or support, underneath you. If the height is sufficient, continue to lie over the bolster. If your head feels considerably lower than your hips, take a blanket folded four times lengthwise (see page 230 for instructions), and place it on top (and down the length) of the bolster.

6. Rest your head to whichever side is more comfortable.

7. Take your hand towel, folded lengthwise in thirds (see page 232 for instructions), and make sure it is wide enough to completely cover your eyes. Place your towel underneath your bottom ear (the one against the bolster) just above the bridge of your nose, so you can breathe, and wrap it around and over your eyes. Let it rest gently above your top (exposed) ear.

8. You can also place an eye pillow just above your exposed ear, on top of the towel.

9. Begin breathing deeply through your nose. At first, lengthen both your inhale and your exhale. As you continue to breathe, experiment with making your exhale longer than your inhale to quiet your mind. If you're following this posture sequence but doing the second sequence in chapter 10, for Anxious Body/Depressed Mind, use 1:1 Breathing instead.

⌒ *Reminder: In rewiring your mind and body, comfort is everything!*

GUIDELINES FOR ADDITIONAL SUPPORT

Softening your neck: If you experience neck pain with your head to the side, cross your forearms and rest your forehead straight down on your forearms so that neither your head nor your neck have to turn.

Supporting your torso: If you are tall, and the blanket folded four times with a lengthwise fold does not cover the length of your torso and head, fold your blanket lengthwise three times so that it is slightly lower, but long enough to support your entire torso and head (fig. 8.2).

Relaxing your feet: If your feet are uncomfortable, place a blanket roll under the ankles. This will allow the feet to flex rather than extend (fig. 8.3, under the ankles). Place the roll wherever the ankles feel tightest (see page 231 for folding and placement instructions for Child's Pose with ankle support). You may need to adjust the blanket roll to be larger (and thus higher) or smaller (lower); your ankles should feel less pressure, so that your feet do not fall asleep. Note that when you support your feet in this way, or add a blanket or two behind your knees (see "Protecting your knees," below), this raises the height of your hips and buttocks. Accordingly, you will want to add an additional blanket or two on top of your bolster to make your torso level (see "Supporting your torso," above).

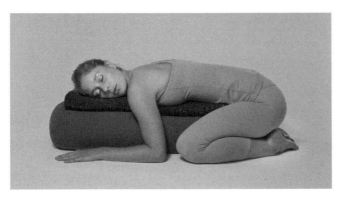

fig. 8.2

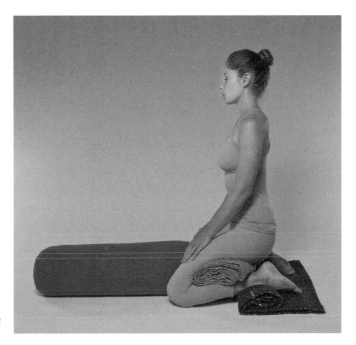

fig. 8.3

Protecting your knees: If you have discomfort in your knees, it may be because of the pressure of your knee bones on the floor beneath you. If you think this is the case, place a soft blanket or towel underneath your kneecaps (and your bolster) to cushion them.

If your knee discomfort feels related to the flexion (bending) in your knees, it may be due to tightness in your quadriceps and knee ligaments, or difficulties with your knee cartilage. If you have this sort of discomfort, fold a blanket four times lengthwise (see page 230 for instructions). Move your body up and off your heels, drawing forward (with your weight on your hands) so that you open the backs of your knees. Using one hand, place the folded blanket tightly in the hollow at the backs of both knees, and then rest your weight back on your heels. When you do so, make sure that the blanket stays at the back of the knees so that it gives you full support (fig. 8.3, behind the knees).

When you add a blanket to support the area behind your knees, you'll need to add two blankets or a small, soft bolster under your torso to make it level with your hips (it's fine if this is approximate rather than exact). You can add height by using one or two

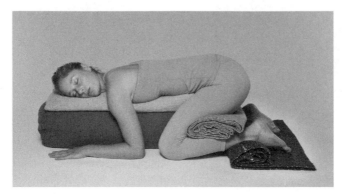

fig. 8.4

blankets folded lengthwise four times or another bolster, cushion, or pillows.

Opening your hips: If you feel tightness in your hips, add a blanket folded (not rolled) lengthwise four times (as you'd do to support your torso, above) behind the knees or place an additional small, soft pillow behind your knees (fig. 8.3). Rest your forearms on the mat next to the bolster. If your elbows do not reach the floor, you can support them (especially the forearm toward which your head turns) with blankets or pillows.

Supporting everything: If you experience discomfort (or less than optimal comfort) in your feet, knees, and hips, add props, as above, to all areas (fig. 8.4). You can experiment by adding more support. See if this alleviates discomfort and builds your body's awareness of the power of support in your practice.

⌒ RECLINING TWIST

Time: 5–30 *minutes on each side*
TRACKS 4–5

Props

- 1 round bolster (or alternative; see page 228)
- 1–2 blankets
- 1 hand towel
- 1 eye pillow

INSTRUCTIONS

1. Place your bolster lengthwise on your mat, just as you did in Child's Pose. If you added blankets on top of your bolster in Child's Pose, remove them now. You will likely not need them here, but you can always add more height later if your body would benefit from it.

2. Sit behind your bolster, as you did in Child's Pose. You'll begin by twisting your torso to the right. Accordingly, sit down with your legs extended to the left, at greater than a right angle (say, at a 110-degree angle) to the bolster (fig. 8.5). Your right hip will touch the shorter side (the width) of the bolster.

3. Fold your legs, with the right leg underneath the left, and your feet pointing to the back of your mat. Once again, make sure that the angle between your thighs and the bolster is greater than a right angle (greater than 90 degrees). This will ensure that your spine can twist comfortably.

4. Fold a blanket lengthwise four times (see page 230 for instructions). Place it between your shins and feet, with the rounded (uniform) edge in toward you (fig. 8.6). If your hips would like more support (more openness), add a second blanket, folded similarly (or half the thickness of the first) between your shins.

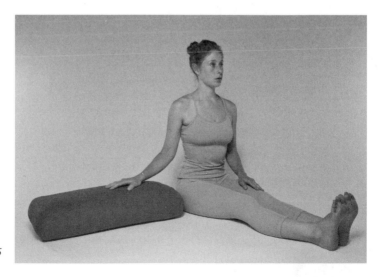

fig. 8.5

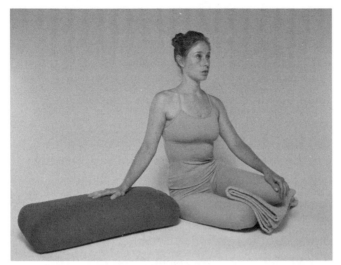

fig. 8.6

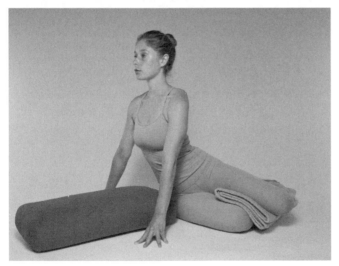

fig. 8.7

5. Remain upright and lengthen your spine as you twist your lower left waist to the right. Face forward so that your upper body is poised to draw down the length of the bolster. Now your feet face the back wall while your torso faces forward, creating a mild spinal twist. Place one hand on either side of the bolster. Sit upright and extend your arms long so that you grow taller. Keep your torso in line with the bolster and maintain the twist in your lower waist and spine (fig. 8.7).

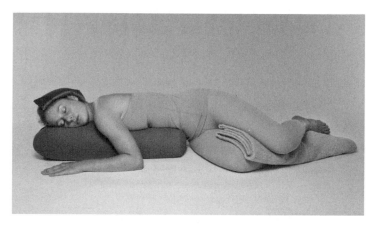

fig. 8.8

6. Inhale and lift your chest and heart area. As you exhale, draw your torso down over the bolster. Rest your head in the same direction (on this side, it would be to the left) as your knees (fig. 8.8).

7. Wrap your eyes with your towel. Place an eye pillow on the left side of your head, leaving your ear uncovered.

8. Rest your forearms on the floor. As in Child's Pose, if your left forearm (when you do this pose on the other side, it would be your right forearm) is elevated above the mat, support it with a blanket.

9. Is your body comfortable? If it isn't, turn to the Guidelines for Additional Support. If it is, breathe deeply through your nose. You have a variety of choices for your breathwork. The speed of your mind, together with your comfort level with the breathing techniques, will determine which breath ratio to choose. If you are most comfortable with simple nasal breathing, practice that. If you'd like to use a slightly longer exhale to calm your mind, you can do so as well. When this is comfortable, you may transition into 1:2 Breathing. Imagine your breath intering any part of your body that needs to let go. Use your breath to help your body relax.

Note that if you are practicing the second sequence in chapter 10 (for Anxious Body/Depressed Mind), but following this chapter's posture sequence, your breath ratio will most likely be 1:1 Breathing, or nasal breathing using your natural breath ratio.

10. Repeat on the other side.

⌐ *Reminder: Your body has the wisdom to tell you what feels comfortable.*

GUIDELINES FOR ADDITIONAL SUPPORT

Supporting your shoulders: If you feel any discomfort in your shoulders or elbows, try supporting the forearm that's on the same side as your knees (on this first side, it would be the left forearm). To do so, use a blanket folded four times or as high as is comfortable (see step 8 above).

Aligning your upper spine and neck: If you feel that your head is much lower than your hips (which will make your torso slope downward toward the front of the bolster), you will need more height on top of the entire length of the bolster. In this case, add a blanket (folded four times) underneath you, until your head is level with your torso. If your chest feels a bit collapsed and it is hard to breathe, add "shoulder pads" (hand towels, folded three times as on page 232) underneath each shoulder.

Taking Stock of How It's Going

At this point in your Restorative Yoga practice, you will transition to face-up poses. In some cases, face-up poses can cause your mind to speed up. How will you know if this happens? First, if the rate of your thoughts accelerates, this pose may be too mentally stimulating for you. Second, a subjective sense of anxiety can creep up on you.

If you feel too active mentally, first make sure that you are breathing in the 1:2 ratio, with the exhale twice as long as the inhale (see page 72 for 1:2 Breathing instructions). If you are already breathing in this ratio and your mind speeds up, or you have difficulty with this breathing ratio, you may find it easier to move on. Your next option is to transition to the neutral restorative poses at the end of this chapter (either Side-Lying Pose or Legs-up-the-Wall Pose). Practice these for a while and then move on to the next pose in this sequence.

INVERSION POSE

Time: 5–10 *minutes*

TRACK 6

PROPS

- 2–3 blankets
- 1 hand towel
- 1 eye pillow
- 1 bolster for weighting, if desired

INSTRUCTIONS

1. Fold one blanket twice (first lengthwise, then widthwise) so it forms a wide and long rectangle (see page 231 for blanket-folding instructions for Inversion Pose). Try one blanket first and see if the height is sufficient for your body. If it isn't, you can stack a second blanket directly on top of the first.

2. Place the blanket(s) on your mat with the rounded, uniform edge facing the back of your mat. Place the blanket(s) on the front half of your mat so that you leave at least half the mat behind you for your shoulders and head.

3. Sit down on the blanket(s), facing the front of your mat, with about 12 inches of blanket behind you. The rest of the blanket(s) will extend forward and off your mat (fig. 8.9).

4. Lie over the blanket(s) so that your upper shoulder blades are grounded on the mat (fig. 8.10). It's important to have your head and the top part of your shoulder blades *on the mat* while the bottom of your shoulder blades and the rest of your body (from your heart area to your feet) are elevated *on the blanket(s)*. The exact placement isn't always easy to get on the first try; you may need to adjust a few times in order to find the best alignment.

5. Draw your arms out from the sides of your body at approximately a 45-degree angle. You can either turn your palms face-up, or rest on the sides of your wrists. If you find it more comfortable, you may also turn your hands over so that your palms face the floor.

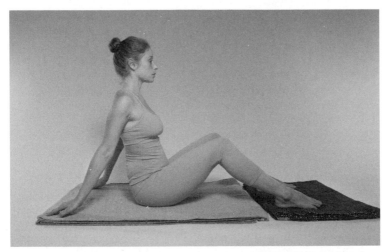

fig. 8.9

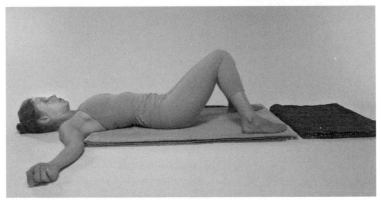

fig. 8.10

6. Start with your knees bent (fig. 8.10). Set the soles of your feet wide, at the outer edges of your mat. Let your knees fall together, and relax your legs.

7. As you breathe, bring your awareness to your head and neck. Make sure that they are comfortable and free of tension.

8. Take a moment to feel how things are going. You are the best judge of your comfort level. You'll be able to tell whether the height of the blanket(s) in this pose is too much for you today or whether it's just right. If it's too much, you will feel active stretching—an exaggerated or forced opening—in your chest and upper spine area. See the "Guidelines for Additional Support" section below to help you adjust for this.

9. Place an eye pillow over your eyes, or on/above your browbone, to further reduce sensory stimulation. If you don't have an eye pillow, use your hand towel instead. You can also use your hand towel, and place your eye pillow on top of it, to further reduce sensory stimulation.

10. Breathe deeply through your nose. If your mind speeds up too much or feels anxious, allow your exhale to be longer than your inhale, or begin 1:2 Breathing. If your mind is balanced or slow, practice 1:1 Breathing. Allow your exhale to take you deeper inward. Keep relaxing your body. Let your thoughts move across the surface of your awareness. When a challenging thought or emotion arises, focus on your breath and your body, and let the thought or emotion pass in its own time.

⌁ *Reminder: The sensation of active stretching is a signal that your body is doing too much and not relaxing.*

Guidelines for Additional Support

Weighting your body: "Weighting" Restorative Yoga poses can feel grounding for people with anxiety or activation, and soothing and supportive for people with depression or lethargy. In Inversion Pose, you can experiment with weighting by placing a bolster, 1–2 blankets folded four times, a pillow, or a cushion either widthwise across your abdomen (see fig. 9.14, page 205) or lengthwise down your body (see fig. 9.5, page 195). If you don't like the feeling of a weight on top of you, just remove it.

Listening to your body: Avoid "pushing" in this pose. Remember that active stretching creates physical tension, which over-engages the sympathetic nervous system and can reinforce negative emotional patterns. Tension also reduces the comfort you will experience in the pose. When you support the body and allow it to open at its own pace, you maximize relaxation. Both your physical flexibility and mental calm will develop faster.

Protecting your shoulders and neck: If you do feel active stretching, lower the height of your blanket by unfolding it so that it is the

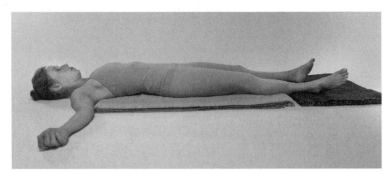

fig. 8.11

same length but twice the width as before (see page 230 for folding instructions).

Supporting your lower back: If you have a tendency to feel tenderness in your lower back, or if you begin to feel strain in this pose when your legs extend straight, bend your knees (fig. 8.10). If you don't typically feel strain in your lower back, you can extend your legs (fig. 8.11). Add another blanket under your feet (the same height as under your torso and legs) to ensure that your entire body is level.

⌒ SIDE-LYING POSE
Time: 5–15 minutes on each side
TRACKS 7–8

PROPS

- 1 round bolster (or alternative; see page 232)
- 3 blankets
- 1 hand towel
- 1 eye pillow

A QUICK WORD ABOUT THIS POSE

If your mind speeds up, you feel anxious, or you have too much physical energy when you are on your back, you can substitute this pose for Relaxation Pose or for Butterfly Pose (discussed in chapter 9). You can also use it as an alternative if Child's Pose isn't comfortable or enjoyable for you.

INSTRUCTIONS

1. Fold one blanket once lengthwise and once widthwise (see page 231 for instructions). Prepare two additional blankets by folding them four times as in the previous poses. They will support your shins and, if needed, the side of your head when you lie down.

2. Sit on your mat on your right side, with your legs folded as they were in Reclining Twist (your right leg will be under your left). Extend the double-folded blanket down your mat with the shorter, rounded side beginning at your waist and the ends extending beyond your head.

3. Place one of the four-folded blankets between your legs, just as you did in Reclining Twist. Keep one of the others handy for possible use underneath your head (fig. 8.12).

4. Slide your right arm down and inside the first blanket; when you are almost lying on your arm, as you'd do if you were going to sleep, fold one edge of the blanket over the top of your extended arm so it creates padding between your outstretched shoulder and the side of your head (fig. 8.13).

5. Many people appreciate an additional four-times-folded blanket between their right shoulder and right ear. Try it and see if it helps support your neck. You can always lower the height of the blanket under your head by half, if you wish.

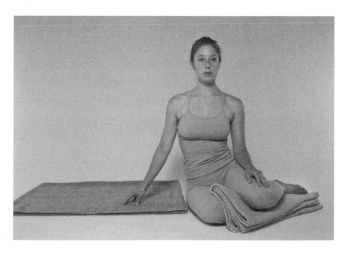

fig. 8.12

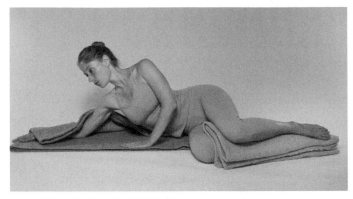

fig. 8.13

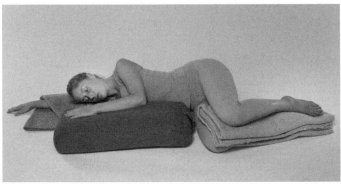

fig. 8.14

6. Bring the bolster in toward your body. Hug it using your left arm (fig. 8.14).

7. As in Child's Pose, you can wrap your eyes with your towel and place an eye pillow on the side of your head (leaving your ear uncovered).

8. Breathe deeply through your nose. If your mind and thoughts are moving fast, let your exhale be longer than your inhale, or move into 1:2 Breathing. If your mind is balanced or slow, lengthen both your inhale and your exhale, and practice 1:1 Breathing instead.

9. Repeat on the other side.

⌢ *Reminder: Remember that these instructions are guidelines, not rules; allow yourself the freedom to adjust your practice in ways that suit you.*

GUIDELINES FOR ADDITIONAL SUPPORT

Protecting your neck: If your neck feels strained in this pose, make sure that you have placed a blanket, folded four times (or, for less height, folded once or twice), under the side of your head, rounded edge in first, for support.

Encountering the unexpected: If your right arm falls asleep, transition onto your other side.

LEGS-UP-THE-WALL POSE

Time: 5–15 minutes

TRACK 9

PROPS

- 2–3 blankets
- 1 hand towel
- 1 eye pillow
- 1 bolster, if desired, for weighting the body

INSTRUCTIONS

1. Bring your mat into the wall, with the short side (width) of the mat flush against the wall.

2. Take a stack of two blankets, folded four times as in the previous poses, and place them next to the mat. As you move, keep your gaze soft and your movements slow, so this transition remains a part of your practice.

3. Sit down with your left hip close to the wall and your knees bent (fig. 8.15).

4. Swing your legs up the wall and lie down in the center of the mat. The first time you do this, it might feel a bit awkward. With practice, the transition will become more fluid.

5. Work your buttocks into the wall. If your hamstrings feel tight, bend your knees and bring your buttocks away from the wall.

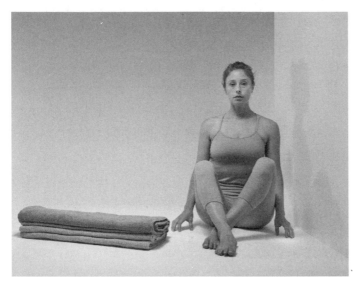

fig. 8.15

6. Bend your knees, walk your feet a little bit down the wall, and lift up your hips. You'll now have space underneath your lower back and buttocks where you can put the blankets for support (fig. 8.16).

7. Place the two four-folded blankets under your hips. Move them an inch or so away from the wall, and even further away if your hamstrings need more space today.

8. If your hamstrings allow, draw your buttocks up and over the blankets or bolster, until they are flush against the wall (fig. 8.17). The blankets will be directly under your buttocks. Your abdomen will slope gently downward toward your heart.

9. Place an eye pillow over your eyes, or on your browbone, to further reduce sensory stimulation and quiet your nervous system. If you don't have an eye pillow, place your folded hand towel over your eyes. You can also use both a hand towel over your eyes, and an eye pillow placed on top.

10. Breathe deeply through your nose. If your mind is active and your thoughts are fast, let your exhale be longer than your inhale or move into 1:2 Breathing. If your mind is balanced or slow (or

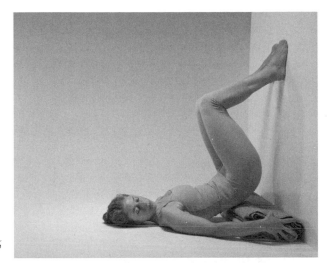

fig. 8.16

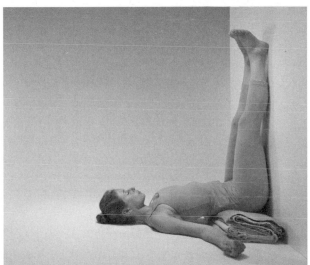

fig. 8.17

you are following the second sequence in chapter 10, for Anxious Body/Depressed Mind), lengthen both your inhale and your exhale and keep a 1:1 breath ratio.

> ⌁ *Reminder: "Weighting" Restorative Yoga poses can be grounding for people with anxiety and soothing for people with depression.*

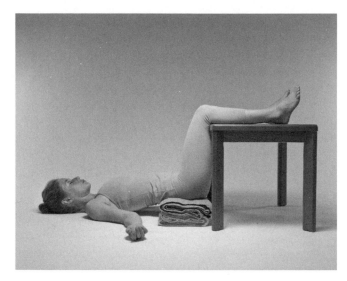

fig. 8.18

GUIDELINES FOR ADDITIONAL SUPPORT

Weighting your body: In Legs-up-the-Wall Pose, as in all the poses, you can experiment with weighting by placing a bolster either widthwise across your body or lengthwise (with the bottom end or width on your abdomen, and the length of the bolster going up the wall against your legs) down your body for a sensation of added support and grounding.

Encountering the unexpected: If your legs fall asleep, come out of the pose.

Adjusting for your hamstrings: If your feet fall asleep, or your hamstrings feel tight at the time of your practice, try this pose with your lower legs supported on a couch, chair, or side table. You can lie down on your back and simply lift your lower legs onto the couch, chair, or side table (fig. 8.18). Make sure, if you try this option, that you place the blankets under your buttocks, and that the height of the table, chair, or couch is enough for your knees to be a little higher than your feet. This prevents strain in the lower back and legs.

Contraindication: It is inadvisable to practice this pose if you are menstruating or pregnant.

FACE-DOWN RELAXATION POSE

Time: 5–15 minutes

TRACK 10

PROPS

- 1 blanket
- 1 eye pillow

INSTRUCTIONS

1. For this pose, we'll fold the blanket in a slightly different way: three times lengthwise so that you have a long, thin blanket about the same length as your mat (see page 231 for instructions). The blanket should be about 6 inches wide, and no higher than three inches tall (fig. 8.19).

2. Lie over the blanket so that it is *under your abdomen,* not under your hips. Ideally, the blanket will fit between your hip bones and your lower ribs. Your lower ribs should be in front of the blanket. Your hip bones should be nearly touching the blanket but a little behind it (fig. 8.20).

3. If your ribs or hip bones are pressing into the blanket, the blanket is too wide. This can cause compression in your lower back. Refold the blanket so that it's narrower and more comfortable.

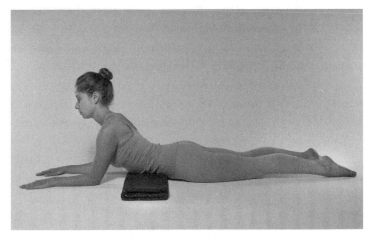

fig. 8.19

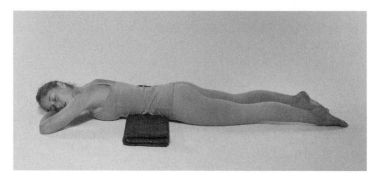

fig. 8.20

4. If the blanket is too wide, refold it once lengthwise, then width-wise, and then fold it in thirds lengthwise (see page 231 for instructions).

5. If your torso is on the longer side, you will want a wider fold. In this case, fold your blanket three times: first lengthwise, then widthwise, then lengthwise in thirds. Place it on your mat with the rounded edge closer to the front of the mat.

6. Lie over the blanket. Make a pillow of your arms or hands and rest your head to either side. If this is uncomfortable on your neck, you can rest your forehead straight down on your hands.

7. If your head is turned to the side, you can place an eye pillow on the side of your head, above your ear. If your head is looking down, you can place an eye pillow on the back of your head or neck.

8. Breathe deeply through your nose. Let your exhale be longer than your inhale or move into 1:2 Breathing. If you are practicing the sequence for Anxious Body/Depressed Mind, use 1:1 Breathing instead.

⌒ *Reminder: The patience and self-care you bring to this practice can extend to your life outside of the practice.*

GUIDELINES FOR ADDITIONAL SUPPORT

Protecting your neck: If you feel neck strain when your head is turned to the side, fold your arms, hold your elbows, and rest your forehead on your hands.

Feel the Difference

Now that you have tried the Anxiety-Balancing Practice, take a few moments to check in with your body and mind. Gauge how the practice has affected you. How does your body feel? Quiet and grounded, very energetic, or somewhere in between? Does your mind feel calmer and more balanced? Or is it still a little racing and worried?

If you feel any agitation or anxiety, try doing some detective work. Is your agitation mental? Ask yourself when your agitation began. Did it happen at the very beginning, in Child's Pose? If so, you may have been unable to breathe well as you rested forward over the bolster. If you think this might be the case, you can place "shoulder pads," or folded hand towels, under each shoulder/pectoral area to raise it a little (see p. 232 for folding instructions). This will open your chest and make your breathing easier. Try it and see. Does your breathing improve? If so, then the discomfort you felt likely means that you needed further support to feel most comfortable.

If your mind became agitated in this Anxiety-Balancing sequence, remember the "hierarchy" of ways in which to address discomfort or anxiety. 1. First, you can add more support to the pose. 2. Then you can change your breath ratio to 1:2 Breathing. 3. If the discomfort persists, you can move on to the next pose in the forward-bending sequence. 4. Finally, you also have the option to change to a neutral restorative pose. If you still feel anxious, you can also use your breath to calm your mind. Simply lengthen your exhale even more than in 1:2 Breathing. This will continue to slow your heart and support relaxation.

Occasionally, the pose itself can be the cause of your discomfort; this may mean that it's best if you leave the pose out of your sequence. Here's an example: for some people, Child's Pose simply doesn't feel comfortable no matter what they try. They may experience agitation, and place towels under the shoulder and pectoral area for support. Yet while they breathe better with this support, and have tried 1:2 Breathing, the agitation persists. This may mean that the pose itself is the culprit. If this happens to you, move on to Reclining Twist and see how that feels. If you encounter similar discomfort there, don't force your body to stay in the forward-bending postures. You can always move on to neutral poses: Inversion Pose, Side-Lying Pose, and Legs-up-the-Wall Pose.

If you do move on from the forward bends, it's always better to transition to neutral restorative poses before switching to back-bending restorative poses. Also, avoid switching back and forth between forward-bending and back-bending postures. This can over-stimulate the nervous system. When you move gradually from forward-bending to back-bending poses via the neutral restorative poses, you minimize the potential for becoming anxious.

It's possible that, even though you perceive yourself to be physically agitated, your body prefers you to be on your back in heart-opening poses. If you experienced discomfort or unrest in the forward-bending postures, consider whether the anxiety you feel stems mostly from your mind, while your body may actually have symptoms of depression. If you think this might be the case, try the first practice in chapter 10 for Depressed Body/Anxious Mind or "Anxious Depression") and see how that works for you.

~9

Depression-Lifting Practice
Energizing Your Body and Mind

THE DEPRESSION-LIFTING PRACTICE IS DESIGNED FOR those with Depressed Body/Depressed Mind those with Depressed Body/Anxious Mind. It features back-bending (face up) restorative poses to open, energize, and uplift your body. If your mind is sluggish or balanced, you will use 1:1 Breathing (see page 48) to keep your mind calm, yet also alert. But if you have an anxious mind, you will use 1:2 breathing (see page 72) to calm your mind and nervous system.

Each time you get ready to practice, take a few moments to check in with yourself and record your mental and physical baselines so you can measure any changes that occur as a result of your practice. Also, you can add brief check-ins between poses to give you a sense of how each pose affects you and, ultimately, which ones will be most beneficial. Always feel free to remain in a pose for the maximum amount of time recommended, or to practice only one or two poses, if that feels best to your body. The practices in this section can be found on tracks 12–21 of the audio download (see page 8). The download offers you a guide to the practice and talks you through the instructions for getting into and modifying each pose. It also gives you auditory cues for regulating your breath and dealing with thoughts and emotions that might arise while you practice.

Depression-Balancing Posture Sequence

TRACKS 12–21

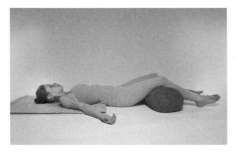

1. *Relaxation Pose*

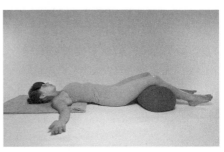

2. *Gentle Backbend Pose*

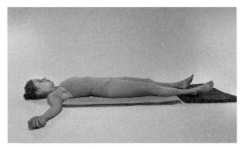

3. *Inversion Pose*

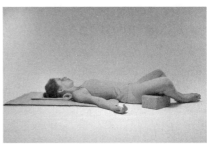

4. *Butterfly Pose*

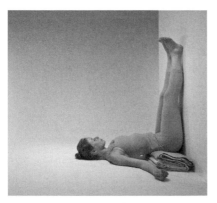

5. *Legs-up-the-Wall Pose*

RELAXATION POSE

Time: 5–10 *minutes*

TRACKS 13–14

PROPS

- 1 round bolster (or alternative; see page 228)
- 1–2 blankets
- 1–3 hand towels
- 1 eye pillow

INSTRUCTIONS

1. Sit down on your mat with your knees bent in front of you and your feet flat on the floor. Place a twice-folded blanket (see page 231 for instructions) on the mat behind you. Have the rounded edge begin at your waist and allow the rest to extend beyond your head. The blanket will support you from the curve of your lower back to the crown of your head, and just beyond. Allow an inch or two between your buttocks and the blanket before you lie over it; this will help support the natural curve of your spine.

2. Place a bolster under your knees and lie down on your back. Take a few breaths, and feel the position of your spine.

3. Take one side of the bolster in each hand so you can move it up or down your legs as you explore how three different placements of the bolster will affect the comfort of your spine. The first place-ment is where your buttocks meet your hamstrings. The second is under the middle of your hamstrings, halfway toward your knees. The third is directly under the backs of your knees. As you try each one breathe, and see which your lower back prefers.

4. Lie down and draw your arms out to a 30- to 45-degree angle from the sides of your body. If it is comfortable for you, place your elbows and hands face up; if it is not comfortable, allow your arms to be halfway between face up and face down (fig. 9.1).

5. You can place an eye pillow over your eyes or on/above your browbone. If you don't have an eye pillow, place your hand towel over your eyes to shut out the light.

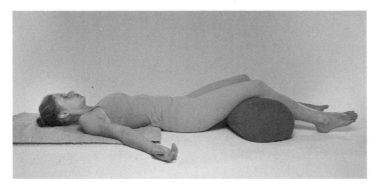

fig. 9.1

6. If you feel any discomfort in this pose, slowly roll onto your side, transition up to sitting, and turn to the Guidelines for Additional Support section below. If you are comfortable, stay where you are.

7. Imagine that you're moving through layers of your body and mind. Breathe deeply and slowly through your nose. Notice where your body might be holding tension. As you inhale, focus on that where tension is; as you exhale, release it. Keep yoking your attention to your breath and your body. After a few minutes, bring your awareness to your mind. Continue your slow and deep breath. Notice your thoughts: are they sluggish or rapid? After some time, try to lengthen both your inhale *and* exhale, and make them equal in length. If you're doing the practice for Depressed Body/Anxious Mind, lengthen just your exhale, or practice 1:2 Breathing.

⌁ *Reminder: In your practice, maintain an evenly hovering attention: an awareness that observes your thoughts, feelings, and sensations without needing to become involved with them.*

GUIDELINES FOR ADDITIONAL SUPPORT

Supporting your spine: If your lower back feels more comfortable in an arched position (which can help with some spinal disc issues), add more support underneath it. Place a second folded blanket on top of the first one (lengthwise down your mat), lining up the rounded edges so that the part under your lumbar spine is even. This will allow for a slightly deeper spinal curve.

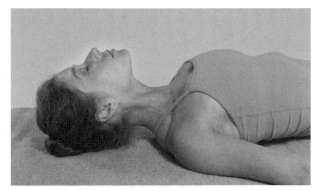

fig. 9.2

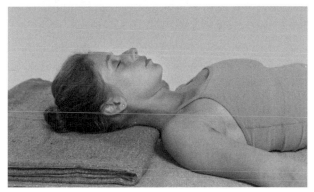

fig. 9.3

Protecting your neck: In Relaxation Pose, as in all the back-bending restorative poses, pay attention to your neck, throat, and breath. If you normally have rounding in your upper spine or shoulders, your neck may hyperextend while you're on your back (fig. 9.2).

If your neck hyperextends, or it is difficult to breathe, or you feel tension in your neck or throat, you may benefit from a blanket folded two to four times under your head (see page 230 for instructions) (fig. 9.3). If the blanket fold feels good to you here, you may wish to use it in all of the back-bending (face-up) Restorative Yoga poses.

If you have a deep cervical curve, your neck might feel unsupported rather than hyperextended when you lie on your back. One way to verify this is to draw one of your hands underneath your neck; if there is an inch or two of blank space underneath, it may feel better with more support. For support, you can experiment with a towel roll under the neck. Fold a hand towel or dish towel in

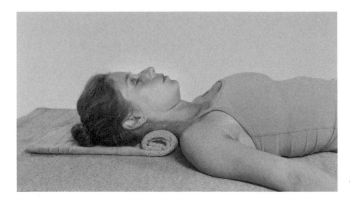

fig. 9.4

half lengthwise and then roll it tightly into a ball (see page 232 for instructions). You can adjust the thickness of the neck roll so that your neck feels supported but not overly so (fig. 9.4). Make sure the roll is not so high that it places pressure on the back of your neck from below. If the neck roll works well for you here, you may wish to use it in each of the successive back-bending Restorative Yoga poses, and also in Legs-up-the-Wall Pose.

If your shoulders naturally tend to round forward when you stand upright (check this using a mirror if you are unsure), you may feel more comfortable with a folded blanket under your head.

Supporting your shoulders: If your shoulders do tend to round forward, they may lift off the floor a little or a moderate amount in most of the back-bending restorative postures. If this happens, you can add "shoulder pads" underneath them for support. To do this, fold two hand towels, each into squares (fold four times to make a square) and place one under each shoulder blade. Experiment with the placement of the hand towels; they can move higher up the spine toward your head, or lower down your spine toward your feet. They can also be moved in toward your spine (closer together) or out away from your spine (farther apart). Feel the difference: if adding the "shoulder pads" and neck support helps relax your shoulders and neck, continue to use them in your other back-bending poses as needed.

Weighting your body: "Weighting" Restorative Yoga poses can feel grounding for people with anxiety or activation, yet soothing and

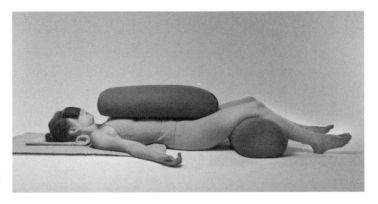

fig. 9.5

supportive for people with depression or lethargy. In Relaxation Pose, you can experiment with weighting by placing a bolster, 1–2 blankets folded four times, a pillow, or a cushion either widthwise across your abdomen or lengthwise down your body (fig. 9.5). If you don't like the feeling of a weight on top of you, just remove it. If you do like it, you can add it in virtually any restorative pose.

GENTLE BACKBEND POSE

Time: 5–30 minutes

TRACKS 15–16

PROPS

- 1 round bolster (or alternative; see page 228)
- 1–4 blankets
- 1 hand towel
- 1 eye pillow

A QUICK WORD ABOUT THIS POSE

In this pose, you will transition to a slightly deeper backbend. Your chest and heart area will lift and expand more than in Relaxation Pose. Self-awareness becomes even more important in helping you gauge your level of physical comfort and your level of mental activation. Both physical discomfort and mental activation are indications that something about the pose (either the level of backbend, your breathing ratio, or the pose itself) needs to be adjusted.

It's possible that raising the height under your upper back in this pose may cause slight physical discomfort. If this happens, remove the fold in your blanket and either practice Supported Relaxation Pose, or move on to the next pose in the sequence. If you have anxiety in your mind, try using the four solutions mentioned earlier: First, use your breathing to manage your anxiety. You can move from 1:1 Breathing to a slightly longer exhale; if this doesn't lessen the anxiety, transition to 1:2 Breathing. Second, if changing your breath has little affect on your discomfort or anxiety, transition to the next pose in this sequence. Third, if that doesn't work, choose a neutral restorative pose (see Inversion Pose, page 175; Side-Lying Pose, page 178; or Legs-up-the-Wall Pose, page 181). Fourth, if you still feel a sense of anxiety or agitation after trying these three solutions, you can choose a forward-bending pose until you feel calmer.

INSTRUCTIONS

1. Fold one blanket twice (first lengthwise, then widthwise) so it forms a wide and long rectangle (see page 231 for blanket-folding instructions).

2. Place the blanket on your mat with the more rounded edge toward you at the front of your mat. Sit down on the mat so that you are facing the blanket. You can kneel on your mat, or sit cross-legged, so that its edge is about 12 inches from your knees or your feet.

3. Take the blanket's edge that is closest to you (the rounded edge) and fold three to four inches of it away from you toward the other edge (fig. 9.6). The blanket will be placed widthwise underneath your body with a good amount of blanket extending behind you to support your head.

4. Lie back over the blanket so that the fold is under your upper spine. The tops of your shoulder blades and your head will be on the mat, while your lower shoulder blades will lift up onto the fold of the blanket. Stretch your arms out just below the level of your

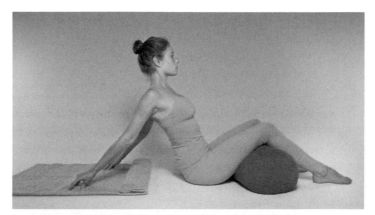

fig. 9.6

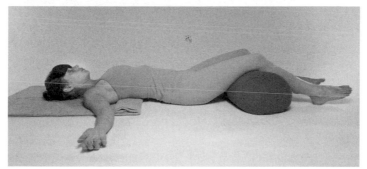

fig. 9.7

heart so that they lie *above the blanket fold,* away from your hips (fig. 9.7). Make sure that the rest of the blanket extends beyond your head and doesn't end abruptly underneath your neck or head.

5. Begin with one fold under your upper back and see how that feels when you are lying down. If you can feel the elevation in your chest, however subtle it may be, then the height of the blanket is sufficient. If you need the fold to be higher in order to feel the elevation, you can fold the blanket over once more. Remember, though: subtle interventions can create the deepest relaxation and have the greatest impact.

6. Place a bolster under your knees, as in Relaxation Pose.

7. You can place an eye pillow over your eyes or on your browbone to further reduce sensory stimulation. If you don't have an eye pillow, place your hand towel, folded lengthwise in thirds, over your eyes to shut out the light.

8. Continue to breathe in and out through your nose, using the breath ratio that's right for you: either 1:1 Breathing to keep your mind balanced and calm, or a longer exhale or 1:2 Breathing to calm your mind more strongly.

⌒ *Reminder: Don't force yourself to fit the practices in this book; give yourself permission to let the practices fit you.*

GUIDELINES FOR ADDITIONAL SUPPORT

Weighting your body: Adding weight on top of your body in restorative postures can feel grounding and balancing for people with anxiety. At the same time, it can feel soothing and supportive for people with depression or lethargy. It's easier to weight your pose when you're on your back. As in Relaxation Pose, experiment with weighting by placing a bolster either widthwise across your abdomen or lengthwise down your body. If you don't like it, you can remove it right away.

Protecting your neck: In Gentle Backbend Pose, as in all the backbending restorative poses, pay attention to your neck, throat, and breath. If you normally have rounding in your upper spine or shoulders when standing or lying down, your neck will most likely hyperextend while you are on your back (see fig. 9.2, page 193).

If your neck hyperextends, you have difficulty breathing, or you feel tension in your neck or throat, you may benefit from a folded blanket under your head (see page 230 for instructions). To prop your head, place the rounded edge of a blanket underneath it (see fig. 9.4, page 194) down almost to where your shoulders begin.

If your neck hyperextends despite placing a blanket under your head, it may be a sign that the elevation under your chest is too high. If this is the case, consider returning to Relaxation Pose, which requires less shoulder support, or moving on to Inversion Pose.

If your neck doesn't hyperextend, but you have a more pronounced curve in your neck, you will need a different sort of neck support. You can assess this by sliding your hand underneath your neck while you're lying down to see whether you feel a lot of space there. If you do, try experimenting with a towel roll under your neck. A hand towel or dish towel, folded in half lengthwise and then rolled down its width (see page 232 for instructions) is ideal for supporting your cervical (neck) spine (see fig. 9.4, page 194). To create more expansion around your chest and heart area, make sure that your arms are extended at a 45-degree angle from your body. If it is comfortable for you to do so, turn your palms up to the ceiling. If this is not comfortable, rest on the outer edge of your hands so that your palms face the sides of your body.

Taking Stock of How It's Going

If you are practicing the Depression-Lifting Sequence in its entirety, the upcoming pose (Inversion Pose) will represent the midpoint of your practice. This means that you can add an extra check-in here to see how your body and mind have received the practice so far. If you have begun to feel anxiety in your mind, you may be closer to the Depressed Body/Anxious Mind emotional type. How can you tell if your mind becomes anxious? Your thoughts may speed up or take on a tone of worry.

On the other hand, your anxiety may be in your body. You may feel a sense of physical agitation and fidgeting, or a subjective sense of being "wired." If this is the case, you may resemble the Anxious Body/Depressed Mind emotional type. This change may be temporary—you may be fluctuating at the moment—or more long-lasting. Either way, you can adapt your practice to these new inner shifts.

If you feel too active mentally, first make sure that you are breathing with a longer exhale, or in the 1:2 ratio, with the exhale twice as long as the inhale (see page 72 for 1:2 Breathing instructions), as you would in the Depressed Body/Anxious Mind Practice in chapter 10. If you are already breathing in this ratio and your mind speeds up, or you have difficulty with this breathing ratio, you may find it easier to move on to the next pose in the sequence. If this does not help, you can transition to the neutral restorative pose at the end of this sequence (Legs-up-the-Wall Pose). Practice these for a while, and then move on to Butterfly Pose, the next pose in this sequence.

INVERSION POSE

Time: 5–10 *minutes*

TRACK 18

PROPS

- 2–3 blankets
- 1 hand towel
- 1 eye pillow
- 1 bolster for weighting, if desired

INSTRUCTIONS

1. Fold one blanket twice (first lengthwise, then widthwise) so it forms a wide and long rectangle (see page 230 for folding instructions). When doing this pose for the first time, try one blanket first and see if the height is sufficient for your body. If it isn't, you can stack a second blanket directly on top of the first.

2. Place the blanket(s) on your mat with the rounded, uniform edge facing the back of your mat. Place the blanket(s) on the front half of your mat so that you leave at least half the mat behind you for your shoulders and head.

3. Sit down on the blanket(s), facing the front of your mat, with about 12 inches of blanket behind you. The rest of the blanket(s) will extend forward and off your mat (fig. 9.8).

4. Lie over the blanket(s) so that your upper shoulder blades are grounded on the mat (fig. 9.9). It's important to have your head and the top part of your shoulder blades *on the mat* while the bottom of your shoulder blades and the rest of your body (from your heart area to your feet) are elevated *on the blanket(s)*. The exact placement isn't always easy to get on the first try; you may need to adjust a few times in order to find the best alignment.

5. Draw your arms out from the sides of your body at approximately a 45-degree angle. You can either turn your palms face up, or rest on the sides of your wrists. If you find it more comfortable, you may also turn your hands over so that your palms face the floor.

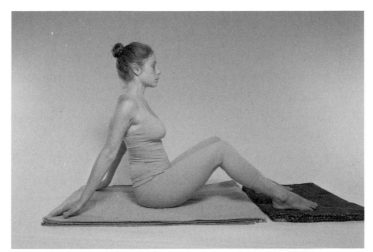

fig. 9.8

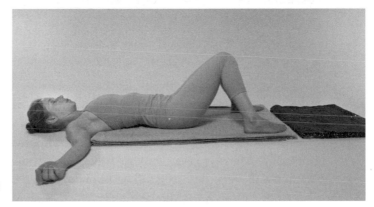

fig. 9.9

6. Start with your knees bent (fig. 9.9). Set the soles of your feet wide, at the outer edges of your mat. Let your knees fall together, and relax your legs.

7. As you breathe, bring your awareness to your head and neck. Make sure that they are comfortable and free of tension.

8. Take a moment to feel how things are going. You are the best judge of your comfort level. You'll be able to tell whether the height of the blanket(s) in this pose is too much for you today, whether it's just right, or whether you will need an additional blanket for more lift. If it's too much, you will feel active stretching—an exaggerated

or forced opening—in your chest and upper spine area. See the "Guidelines for Additional Support" section below to help you adjust for this.

9. Place an eye pillow over your eyes, or on/above your browbone, to further reduce sensory stimulation. If you don't have an eye pillow, use your hand towel instead. You can also use your hand towel, and place your eye pillow on top of it.

10. Breathe deeply through your nose. If your mind is sluggish, depressed, or balanced, practice 1:1 Breathing. If your mind speeds up too much or feels anxious, allow your exhale to be longer than your inhale, or begin 1:2 Breathing.

> Reminder: The sensation of active stretching is a signal that your body is doing too much and not relaxing.

GUIDELINES FOR ADDITIONAL SUPPORT

Weighting your body: In my clinical experience, "weighting" Restorative Yoga poses can feel grounding for people with anxiety or activation, and soothing and supportive for people with depression or lethargy. In Inversion Pose, you can experiment with weighting by placing a bolster, 1–2 blankets folded four times, a pillow, or a cushion either widthwise across your abdomen or lengthwise down your body. If you don't like the feeling of a weight on top of you, just remove it.

Listening to your body: Avoid "pushing" in this pose. Remember that active stretching creates physical tension, which over engages the sympathetic nervous system and can reinforce negative emotional patterns. Tension also reduces the comfort you will experience in the pose. When you support the body and allow it to open at its own pace, you maximize relaxation. Both your physical flexibility and your mental calm will develop faster.

Protecting your shoulders and neck: If you do feel active stretching in your chest, shoulders, or neck, lower the height of your blanket by unfolding it so that it is the same length but twice the width as before.

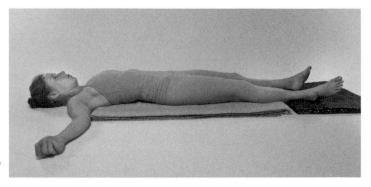

fig. 9.10

Supporting your lower back: If you have a tendency to feel tenderness in your lower back, or if you begin to feel strain in this pose when your legs extend straight, bend your knees (fig. 9.9, page 201). If you don't typically feel strain in your lower back, you can extend your legs (fig. 9.10. If you do extend your legs, add another blanket under your feet (the same height as under your torso and legs) to ensure that your entire body is level.

BUTTERFLY POSE

Time: 5–15 minutes
TRACK 19

PROPS

- 1 round bolster (or alternative; see page 228)
- 1–2 blankets
- 1 hand towel, folded lengthwise
- 1 eye pillow

INSTRUCTIONS

1. Sit on your mat toward the front, with your legs extended straight out ahead of you. Place one or two blankets, folded lengthwise and then widthwise, behind you on the mat. Align the rounded (uniform) edge of the blanket(s) with the curve of your spine (fig. 9.11). This blanket placement is the same as for Relaxation Pose, but twice the height (see page 230). It also reverses the direction of

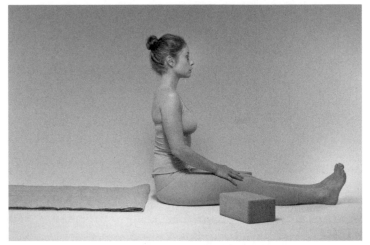

fig. 9.11

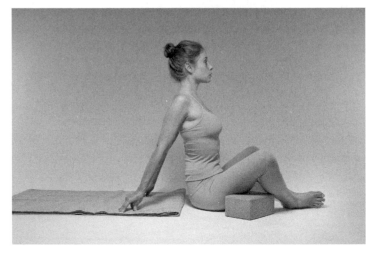

fig. 9.12

the blankets in Inversion Pose. Leave a couple of inches of space between your buttocks and the edge of the blanket.

2. Bend your knees and bring the soles of your feet together, with your knees out toward the sides of your mat in a butterfly position. Place blocks or cushions beneath your thighs at a right angle (fig. 9.12).

3. Lie back over the blanket(s) (fig. 9.13).

4. Keep in mind that your inner thighs should be relaxed and not actively stretching; active stretching will stimulate your mind and

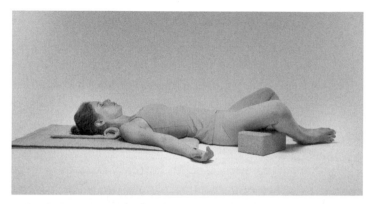

fig. 9.13

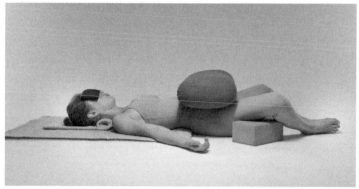

fig. 9.14

brain. For more thigh support, place the blocks farther up your thighs (toward your hips). If you need less support, the blocks can be moved a little toward your knees. It's easier to tell how much support your inner thighs need when you lie down.

5. Place an eye pillow over your eyes or on your browbone to reduce sensory stimulation. If you don't have an eye pillow, put your hand towel over your eyes.

6. Breathe deeply through your nose. If your mind speeds up or feels anxious, allow your exhale to be longer than your inhale, or begin 1:2 Breathing. If your mind feels balanced or slow, practice 1:1 Breathing.

Reminder: Welcome thoughts, emotions, and impulses as a natural part of your practice. Acknowledge them as you breathe in, and release them as you breathe out.

GUIDELINES FOR ADDITIONAL SUPPORT

Weighting your body: In Butterfly Pose, as in all the poses, you can experiment with weighting by placing a bolster either widthwise across your abdomen (fig. 9.14) or lengthwise down your body for a sensation of added support and grounding. If you don't like the feeling of weight on top of you, just remove it. If you do like it, you can add it to virtually any restorative pose.

Supporting your head: In Butterfly Pose, as in Relaxation Pose and the other back-bending restorative poses, pay attention to your neck, throat, and breath. If it's difficult to breathe, or you feel tension in your neck or throat, you would benefit from a blanket fold under your head. If you have rounding in your upper spine or shoulders, your neck will most likely hyperextend while you are on your back (see fig. 9.2, page 193). To support your head, place the rounded edge of a blanket under your head (see fig. 9.4, page 194).

Supporting your shoulders: If you have used "shoulder pads" for support in the back-bending poses above, you can do so here.

LEGS-UP-THE-WALL POSE

Time: 5–15 minutes
TRACK 20

PROPS

- 2–3 blankets
- 1 hand towel
- 1 eye pillow
- 1 bolster, if desired, for weighting the body

INSTRUCTIONS

1. Bring your mat to the wall, with the short side (width) of the mat flush against the wall.

2. Take a stack of two blankets, folded four times (see page 230 for folding instructions). Place them next to your mat.

3. Sit down with your left hip close to the wall and your knees bent (fig. 9.15).

4. Swing your legs up the wall and lie down in the center of the mat. The first time you do this, it might feel a bit awkward. With practice, the transition to bringing your legs up the wall will become more fluid.

5. Work your buttocks into the wall. If your hamstrings feel tight, you can bend your knees and bring your buttocks slightly away from the wall.

6. Bend your knees, walk your feet a little bit down the wall, and lift up your hips. You'll now have space underneath your lower back and buttocks where you can put the blankets for support (fig. 9.16).

7. Place the two four-folded blankets under your hips. Move them an inch or so away from the wall, and even further away if your hamstrings need more space today.

8. If your hamstrings allow, draw your buttocks up and over the blankets or bolster, until they are flush against the wall (fig. 9.17). The blankets will be directly under your buttocks. Your abdomen will slope gently downward toward your heart.

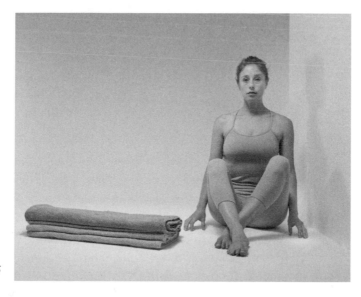

fig. 9.15

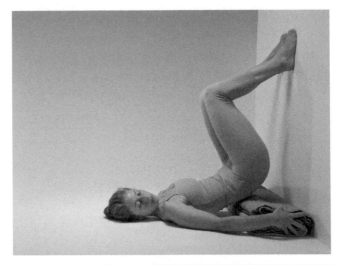

fig. 9.16

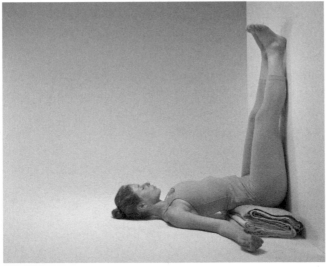

fig. 9.17

9. Place an eye pillow over your eyes, or on your browbone, to further reduce sensory stimulation and quiet your nervous system. If you don't have an eye pillow, place your folded hand towel over your eyes. You can also use both a hand towel over your eyes, and an eye pillow placed on top.

10. Breathe deeply through your nose. If your mind is active and your thoughts are fast, let your exhale be longer than your inhale or move into 1:2 Breathing. If your mind is balanced or slow (or

you are following the second sequence in chapter 10, for Anxious Body/Depressed Mind), lengthen both your inhale and your exhale and keep a 1:1 Breathing ratio.

∽ *Reminder: The subtle practices can create the deepest relaxation and have the greatest impact.*

Guidelines for Additional Support

Weighting your body: In Legs-up-the-Wall Pose, as in all the poses, you can experiment with weighting by placing a bolster either widthwise across your body or lengthwise (with the bottom end or width on your abdomen, and the length of the bolster going up the wall against your legs) down your body for a sensation of added support and grounding.

Encountering the unexpected: If your legs fall asleep, come out of the pose and try Side-Lying Pose.

Adjusting for your hamstrings: If your feet fall asleep, or your hamstrings feel tight at the time of your practice, try this pose with your lower legs supported on a couch, chair, or side table. You can sit on the floor facing the couch or side table, lie down, and simply lift your lower legs onto the top of the table (fig. 9.18). Make sure,

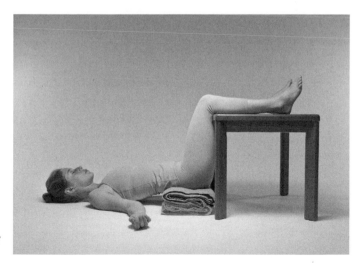

fig. 9.18

if you try this option, that you place the blankets under your buttocks, and that the height of the table or couch is enough for your
knees to be a little higher than your feet. This prevents strain in the
lower back and legs.

Contraindication: It is inadvisable to practice this pose if you are
menstruating or pregnant.

Feel the Difference

Now that you have tried the Depression-Lifting Practice, take a
few moments to check in with your body and mind. How does
your body feel? Rejuvenated, restored, or more open? Now let's do
a quick mental check-in. Does your mind feel more energized yet
still balanced? Or is it racing?

Sometimes physical discomfort can highlight a habitual pattern
of carrying tension in your body. This kind of discomfort eases with
time, and as you allow the breath to move through your body. If
discomfort persists for more than a couple of minutes, or deepens,
it's time to take action. You can be an emotional detective here and
ask yourself what sort of agitation you're feeling—physical or mental—and when it began. Is it physical? If so, did it start with the
first pose: Relaxation Pose? The increased sense of agitation may
be related to physical discomfort. See if you can determine whether
the discomfort is in your back or your neck. Then you know you
can support these areas more fully next time.

If activation occurs not in your body but in your mind, ask yourself when it started. Did it begin with the first pose: Relaxation
Pose? If so, this might be because you don't currently have the kind
of depression that involves both the body and mind. Even though
you have diagnosed your emotional type as Depressed Body/De-
pressed Mind, you may actually have agitation in your mind (or the
potential to generate mental anxiety). This means that you may be
closer to the "Anxious Depression" emotional type. Try the first
practice in chapter 10, for balancing Anxious Depression, to see
whether it works better for you. If so, you don't need to change

positions unless you wish to. You can simply begin 1:2 Breathing (see page 72 for instructions) to calm the agitation in your mind.

If, on the other hand, you don't have a uniformly depressed mind and body but your body is agitated, you may have "Depressed Anxiety," or the Anxious Body/Depressed Mind emotional type. This means that your body has symptoms of anxiety while your mind has signs of depression. If this is the case, the second practice in chapter 10, "Anxious Body/Depressed Mind," for balancing Depressed Anxiety, may work better for you.

Mixed Anxiety and Depression Stabilizing Practices

THE PREVIOUS TWO CHAPTERS OFFERED YOU PRACTICES for uniform anxiety (anxiety in both body and mind) and uniform depression (depression in both body and mind). At times, however, your emotional picture may not be that simple. What if you don't have "straightforward" anxiety or depression but a mixture of the two? For example, even if you have physical and mental symptoms of anxiety, you may still experience depression (in either body or mind) on occasion. Conversely, even if you have a more linear depression in body and mind, you can still experience symptoms of anxiety in either one at times. This means that occasionally you dip your toe into the waters of another emotional type.

Perhaps you don't occasionally dip your toe in but swim regularly in the ocean of mixed anxiety and depression; this means that you have symptoms of both *at the same time, most of the time.* This occurs in two more emotional types, each of which involves a mixture of anxiety and depression. The two practices offered in this chapter target these two emotional types.

Take a few moments in a quiet space to check in and assess yourself before you practice. This helps you be more attuned to variations or fluctuations in your mind and body. These fluctuations are more common if you already have a mixture of anxiety and depression.

Depressed Body/Anxious Mind: Energizing the Body and Calming the Mind

The first practice, for "Anxious Depression," is designed to help when you have physical symptoms of depression (such as lethargy or slowness) but mental symptoms of anxiety (racing thoughts and worry). This practice uses the back-bending restorative sequence to rejuvenate your physical energy and reverse the Closed Heart Syndrome of depression. It also includes 1:2 Breathing to keep your mind balanced and regulated, and to prevent it from speeding up.

If your emotional detective work leads you to conclude that you have the Depressed Body/Anxious Mind emotional type, use the sequence of depression-lifting postures in chapter 9. At the same time, to address your mental symptoms of anxiety, you'll practice the breathwork ratio for anxiety, which is either a longer exhale, or 1:2 Breathing (see page 72 for instructions). Make sure that you practice mindfully and with awareness, so that you note any mental or physical changes. If at any time during the practice you begin to feel anxious, you can adjust your practice. First, be sure that you are using 1:2 Breathing, or an exhale that is longer than your inhale. If the anxious feeling persists, you can transition to the "neutral" Restorative Yoga poses such as Side-Lying Pose or Legs-up-the-Wall Pose. Now, to begin your sequence, turn to the Depression-Lifting Practice.

Anxious Body/Depressed Mind: Calming the Body and Energizing the Mind

The second practice in this chapter is designed for the opposite type of mixed anxiety and depression: "Depressed Anxiety." This practice is geared toward people who have the type of emotional imbalance in which the body displays anxiety or agitation, while the mind exhibits depression or lethargy. This practice uses the Restorative Yoga sequence for anxiety, which consists mostly of forward-bending poses to ground and calm your body. It also uses 1:1 Breathing to keep your mind energized and lift you out of the mental fog that often occurs in depressed anxiety.

If you feel that you have the Anxious Body/Depressed Mind emotional type, turn to the Anxiety-Balancing Practice in chapter 8, where you will find the forward-bending restorative sequence for anxiety. To address your mental symptoms of depression, you'll practice the breathwork ratio for depression in the mind, which is 1:1 Breathing (see page 48 for instructions). If at any time during this practice you feel too physically tired or "overly grounded," transition to the neutral restorative poses such as Side-Lying Pose or Legs-up-the-Wall Pose. If you feel stirrings of anxiety in your mind, move from 1:1 Breathing to an exhale that is longer than your inhale. If the mental anxiety persists, use 1:2 Breathing instead. Now, to begin your sequence, turn to the Anxiety-Balancing Practice.

Epilogue

THE TRADITION OF YOGA RECOGNIZES EMOTIONAL BALANCE as an essential ingredient in true happiness. One of my favorite texts from India's vast body of spiritual literature is the Bhagavad Gita, or "Song of God." The Gita, which makes up approximately seven hundred verses of the hundred-thousand-verse Mahabharata epic, takes place on a battlefield on the eve of war. Arjuna, the protagonist, is caught between two *dharmas*, or duties: should he be a warrior or a family member? His dharma as a warrior requires him to fight against and potentially kill both his grandfather and his guru. His duty as a family member prohibits him from fighting his loved ones. Conflicted, he begs Lord Krishna, who is also his cousin, to release him from battle.

Arjuna is in emotional turmoil: anxious and afraid, but also depressed and helpless. He makes a strong case for not fighting. He wonders how killing can possibly be spiritual. He questions how it can be right to kill his loved ones. Isn't it better to let go of his duty as a warrior? In the powerful dialogue (and instruction on yoga) that ensues, Krishna answers that Arjuna's duty as a warrior eclipses all his other obligations.

Near the end of the Gita, Krishna tells Arjuna that there are three kinds of happiness. The first is called *sattvic:* it is based on *sattva*, a quality of luminosity, wisdom, and joy. The process of developing sattvic happiness is both difficult and humbling. It arises from long dedication to self-study, and from the development of mental and emotional equanimity. It denies the ego but feeds the deepest self, or soul. Krishna says that as we first embark on our spiritual journey and begin the work of examining and shifting our patterns, sattvic happiness can taste like poison. Yet with diligent practice and maturation, it becomes sweet and nourishing, like nectar.

The second kind of happiness is *rajasic:* it arises from *rajas,* which means it depends upon cultivating external image, acquiring power over others, grasping for outcomes, and pursuing the fulfillment of desires. This outer-directed rajasic happiness has the flavor of chronic agitation and anxiety. Because rajas drives us to be active and accomplish things constantly, it masquerades as hard work. It gratifies the ego but starves the soul. The satisfaction of rajas is short-lived; as soon as we've realized one goal, we're captivated by the allure of the next. As Krishna warns, this kind of happiness may taste sweet at first, but inevitably turns bitter and toxic.

The third kind of happiness is *tamasic:* it stems from *tamas,* which refers to the short-term satisfaction of giving up the search for self-awareness and evading the work of emotional balance. Tamasic happiness seduces us to withdraw from the world, and causes indolence, avoidance, and sleep. Tamasic happiness echoes inertia and depression. It may result in the momentary sense of relief that stems from avoidance, yet quickly morphs into suffering. Krishna tells us that tamasic happiness is poisonous almost from beginning to end.

The Gita takes place on the cusp of a mythical battle, which evokes our epic struggle for emotional and spiritual evolution. Arjuna's challenge lies in discerning which duty to honor: householder or warrior. Ours lies in deciding whether to stay in our comfort zone or do battle in order to evolve. While our challenges may differ, we can all relate to Arjuna's dilemma. When faced with painful emotions and difficult life passages, we too may yearn to give up the fight. We may want to avoid the potential conflict and loss that come with self-examination. Yet at heart, we are spiritual warriors.

Committing to the spiritual journey means that, like Arjuna, we may have to "kill" along the way. We may need to let go of parts of ourselves that no longer serve us, no matter how attached we've been to them. We may have to sacrifice the stories and patterns that once defined but no longer nourish us.

We are born with the ability to be emotionally balanced. Our challenge is to recognize the poisonous taste that comes at the journey's onset *not* as an indication that something is wrong, but as an essential stepping-stone on the path to true happiness. Our challenge is to stick with the process, even when we're in doubt of the outcome.

The path to emotional balance is not direct or predictable. It is serpentine, and filled with seemingly impossible tasks. As in all mythic quests, however, these tasks come with unexpected help and hidden rewards. When we connect with our minds and bodies, we can empathize and connect more with others. When we identify our emotional experiences as *not* us, we can encounter the wisdom and balance that *are.*

On the path to emotional balance, we realize that anxiety and depression have something in common with happiness and equanimity. Like all other states of awareness, they come and they go. We will find emotional balance, lose it, and find it, over and over again. We will come to see that the value of the journey doesn't lie in achieving a permanent state of emotional balance. Rather, in the finding and losing of emotional balance, we draw closer to one of the primary goals of yoga therapy: observing and calming the fluctuations of experience that veil our deepest selves.

When we rewire our emotional patterns, we rediscover the art of emotional transformation and inspire others to do the same. And our mindful journey toward sattvic happiness, in the end, reveals its nectar: the wiring we may have thought was confined to our own emotional systems transcends the borders of our imagination. It is actually part of a greater emotional network that connects us with all living things.

ACKNOWLEDGMENTS

I OWE A GREAT DEBT OF GRATITUDE TO MANY PEOPLE. Linda Loewenthal of David Black Literary Agency is a woman of surprising talents: an extraordinary agent, mindful tigress, longtime yogini, and true friend. I am deeply grateful for her support through every stage of this book's development. The Shambhala team includes my editor, Katie Keach, who first envisioned the project, patiently reworked it with me, and gave me time to find my voice. Lenny Jacobs helped with the vision and supported me all the way through. Eden Steinberg and Chloe Foster formed an editorial sandwich, with Eden helping out toward the beginning and Chloe toward the end. Sara Bercholz embodied grace and mindfulness in both the restorative photos and the beautiful cover shot. Thibault Fagonde conveyed the restful yet dynamic qualities of Restorative Yoga in his inspiring photographs.

My brother, Stefan Forbes, interrupted his screenwriting to lend this book his award-winning journalistic expertise, fraternal reinforcement, and tough love. Even when his feedback was at its most critical or began with "WHY, WHY, *WHY* DO YOU ALWAYS," I learned from him. His suggestions were at all times constructive and often hilarious. Without his input, this book would not have matured.

My father, Allan Forbes, Jr., saw in me the makings of a yoga teacher, and encouraged (read: badgered) me to teach. He got involved in my yoga community. He instilled in me a stubborn conviction that I could do anything I set my mind to. Years ago, this meant becoming the only girl on my Little League team, and Dad continues to inspire me in countless ways.

Angelo Cali, my father's best friend for over fifty years, advised me in a letter in 2004 to write about yoga *and* psychology. I had absolutely no idea what he was talking about and filed his letter away, only to retrieve it years later as I was penning my first Yoga Journal article on that very topic. Ange was a visionary and, like my father, saw people clearly. I will always be grateful to him for his guidance and interest in my work.

Edwin Bryant, my dharma brother, saw the seeds of this book in a talk I gave at Harvard Medical School's "Meditation in Psychotherapy" conference in 2006. I'm thankful for Edwin's abiding friendship and our animated discussions about the intersection between yogic philosophy and psychology.

Many dear friends and colleagues have inspired me through their groundbreaking work: Gary Kraftsow, Leslie Kaminoff, Judith Hanson Lasater, Nicolai Bachman, Scott Blossom, Larry Payne, Edwin Bryant, and Patricia Walden for her skill in the therapeutic applications of yoga. I am also grateful to many of the founding members of the Institute for Meditation in Psychotherapy, who have helped the field of psychotherapy develop and whom I consider to be my mentors: Chris Germer, Bill Morgan, Susan Morgan, Susan Pollak, Stephanie Morgan, Janet Surrey, Paul Fulton, Ron Siegel, and Sara Lazar, among others.

Garrett (Dinabandhu) Sarley, Ila Sarley, Rasmani Orth, and Grace Welker of Kripalu understood and supported my vision from the very beginning. The first time I taught there, they welcomed me with open arms. They encouraged my vision and brought to Kripalu countless workshop participants who influenced the direction of my work.

Mark Harrington and Tavia Patusky of Healthworks Fitness Centers played a key role in my professional development since I moved to Boston in 2000. Years ago, Mark and Tavia agreed to purchase bolsters and blankets for a mystery class called "Restorative Yoga." They took a chance because at the time, no one else in the Boston area offered a Restorative Yoga class. I am grateful to Tavia and Mark for their trust, and for making Healthworks a "training hospital" for my annual teacher trainings.

The extraordinary staff at *Yoga Journal* has consistently supported me. They've invited me to their conferences year after year, where I have been able to refine my work with some amazing students and colleagues. Special thanks go to my dear friends Dayna Macy and Elana Maggal, who were there when it all began.

Sat Bir Khalsa and Roger Cole offered their expertise to the research and sleep-related sections of this book, respectively. My University of Chicago master's thesis chair, Justin Miller is the best professor and staunchest supporter of original thinking I've ever had. My pre- and post-doctoral supervisors, M. Mark McKee and John Glennon taught me to look, listen, and think outside the box.

I am indebted to the excellent editors and readers who have had a hand in this book's making, including: Laraine Henner, Linda Sparrowe, Rebecca Steinitz, Edwin Bryant, Fiona Akhtar, Robyn Long, Diana Young, and Christine Rahimi. Several people deserve further thanks for reading the book in its difficult early stages and for somehow refraining from condemnatory judgments on my character or intelligence: Kelly McGonigal, Lucy Arrington, Dayna Macy, Brian Mahoney, and Kathy Hartsell.

The Elemental Yoga community in Boston and throughout the world is an integral part of this book and of my heart. This growing community has offered me warm welcome, yogic mindfulness, and constructive feedback. Special thanks go to each of my teacher training classes, with whom I have played, explored, and engaged in our system of yoga therapeutics in a meaningful and nourishing way.

Writing a book can cause fluctuations in emotional imbalance. I am grateful to the many people who offered me emotional support. Hi-Rise Bakery in Cambridge provided sustenance throughout the last fifteen months of highs and lows, and never once questioned me for ordering "ice tea, no ice." Catherine Weser of One Life has been a wise mentor and spiritual teacher for several years. My family and friends sacrificed a great many days, evenings, holidays, and vacations to support me during the writing of this book. Only on rare occasions did they complain of neglect or comment, "But I thought the final due date was *last month.*" They exhibited great patience with my unavailability, and yet wholeheartedly embraced me each time I resurfaced.

Thanks also go to Wendelin Scott for coining the phrase, "Sudden Repulsion Syndrome." And one last bit of consolation for O., who saw himself in every anecdote. I promise: that's *not* you in chapter 4!

APPENDIX A
Frequently Asked Questions

As you practice Restorative Yoga, questions can arise. It's natural to wonder whether you are "doing it right." Just so you know, it's normal to take weeks, or even months, to determine the combination of breathwork and poses that works best for you. During this assimilation period, you may have questions about the practice. Here I'll share with you the answers to questions I encounter most often while teaching.

Q: Can I practice Restorative Yoga even if I'm not in shape?

A: Anyone can practice Restorative Yoga, regardless of age, shape, or physical condition. The poses are designed to be comfortable, so let comfort be your guide. If you're uncomfortable, try using more props or support. Also consider moving on to the next option in your sequence or experimenting with other poses.

Q: Can I practice Restorative Yoga if I have a medical condition?

A: If you have a physical condition, such as lymphedema, eye or vision problems, or other medical issues, consult your doctor before beginning this practice. Some of the poses are not safe for certain medical conditions. Take time to explain Restorative Yoga, or show pictures of the poses, to your health practitioner so that he or she can give you the most informed answer possible.

Q: What if I don't have a yoga mat or traditional props? Can I practice without props?

A: Not having a yoga mat or proper blankets won't interfere with your practice. Appendix B, "Prop Resource Guide," offers prop alternatives that you will likely have in your home.

Q: What happens if I fall asleep during Restorative Yoga?

A: Falling asleep during the practice is common. If this happens, it may mean that you have accumulated some "sleep debt" and need the extra sleep. If you practice at times of the day when you ordinarily feel sleepy, such as midmorning or mid- to late-afternoon, consider switching to another time of day. Early morning, late afternoon, and early evening are all good times to practice, when your sleep-wake rhythms are less likely to interfere with staying awake.

Q: What do I do if I'm too anxious to lie still and relax?

A: If the stillness of Restorative Yoga is difficult at first, you have options. First, you can practice after physical exertion or exercise (such as an active yoga class or cardiovascular exercise, weight training, or other activities). This sometimes lessens the intensity of any restlessness you may feel. If you experience anxiety while reclining in restorative postures, you can also practice them for limited periods of time. Choose the restorative pose that feels easiest to you and practice it for two to five minutes. Try this for several weeks. You can gradually begin to increase the length of time you spend in your favorite pose. Eventually—and how long it takes to get to this point isn't important—you will be able to sustain a twenty-minute, thirty-minute, or even sixty-minute practice without taking a break.

Q: What do I do if my mind is anxious and activated but I can't seem to lengthen my exhale?

A: If it's hard to make your exhale longer than your inhale, try not to worry. Know that just breathing in and out through your nose naturally makes your exhale a little longer. It takes time to get used to breathing differently. You'll find that with self-compassion and patience, your capacity to regulate your breath will grow.

Q: What if the sequence I've tried is not working?

A: If something doesn't work right away, make a note of it and add a dose of compassion. You can also become a yoga detective, and remain curious. If it didn't work, there's a good reason why. With some patience, you'll hit on a combination that works well for you. If you can remain neutral and inquiring, you'll develop the "emotional muscles" that build equanimity in the midst of diversity. Then difficulty will become a part of your practice rather than an obstacle to it.

Q: What if I'm not choosing the poses—or getting into them—correctly?

A: It's understandable to be concerned that you are not picking the right poses, not doing the poses correctly, or not "getting it right." The most important guide is comfort, which deepens relaxation. If you are used to moderate to intense discomfort, or if you have been living with physical discomfort for a long time, it might not at first be apparent to you that your body is physically uncomfortable in a posture. Don't be concerned; your sense of what feels ease-ful will grow and evolve with time. As you develop the capacity to relax more and more, you will be able to create greater comfort each time you practice.

When practicing, you will also find it helpful to use one of your best inner tools: your capacity to observe yourself, and the fluctuations in your mind and body, with neutrality and compassion. Neutrality may come first: if you've struggled to find emotional balance throughout your life, you've probably been critical of yourself in the process. Like many people, you may have wondered more than once what's "wrong" with you. Sometimes this will come up during your practice. If it does, observe it with neutralilty. Acknowledge it as part of your practice without getting caught up in it. Then gradually, you can practice self-compassion. The key thing to remember is that the qualities of your practice are more important than the results. Your sense of self-compassion, commitment to practicing, dedication to self-awareness, and body awareness all support the practice. They are more essential than either precision or performance.

Q: *What if strong feelings or memories arise during my practice? What do I do with them?*

A: The keys here are deepening your breath and cultivating a neutral attitude toward your memories, emotions, and experiences. Cultivating neutrality is a difficult, yet essential part of changing your patterns. As you now know, negative thoughts can resonate throughout your mind and body. Their emotional charge usually affects your nervous system and causes a shift in your hormones, including stress hormones. In other words, judging yourself is stressful to your system. When feelings arise, breathe through them. You will notice, in time, that they come and go in a natural, organic way.

Q: *Is there an ideal time of day when I should practice?*

A: It's important to practice as regularly as you can. If you have only one time of day available, that's fine. However, your practice may be more challenging in midmorning or mid- to late-afternoon, when you're more likely to fall asleep. Ideal times for practice are during transition times, such as in the early morning before going to work (you might choose to practice only one or two poses, or practice for a shorter length of time) or upon returning home from work. Late at night, before sleep, is also optimal and can help with insomnia.

Q: *Where can I find more information on yoga therapy?*

A: For information on the growing field of yoga therapy, visit www. iayt.org, the official website of the International Association of Yoga Therapists. You can use the site to search for a yoga therapist in your area, read about current research and clinical practice in yoga therapy, or learn more about the process of yoga therapy.

Q: *Can I schedule a yoga therapy session with you?*

A: Typically, the yoga therapists at the Center for Integrative Yoga Therapeutics in Boston have a full roster. You may check our website for more information (http://www.elementalyoga.com/teacher-training/center-for-integrative-yoga-therapeutics/). Since we cannot provide referrals to yoga therapists outside the Boston area, please contact the International Association of Yoga Therapists (www. iayt.org) for a referral to a yoga therapist near you.

Q: What is the purpose of weighting the poses? Can any pose be weighted?

A: Adding weight to a pose (in the form of a soft bolster or blanket) seems to give practitioners an additional sense of grounding, support, and calm. It also helps with the process of drawing awareness inward. You can use weighting in both forward-bending and back-bending restorative practices. You can weight virtually any pose, though some (such as Reclining Twist and Child's Pose) may be more *practically* difficult to weight than others. We encourage you to experiment with the amount of weight and with creative ways to place it when you practice. Weighting can also be used on top of the feet and shins for restless legs.

Q: Is there an optimal way to incorporate Restorative Yoga into my existing yoga routine or into my workout routine?

A: Yes. If you already practice yoga and would like to add Restorative Yoga to your routine, try choosing one or two poses at the end of your routine to deepen your *savasana,* or final relaxation. You can add it after weight-lifting, running, or biking, right after you've done any stretching you might do. If you feel tired or physically ill, you can add a restorative pose (such as a back-bending pose to increase physical energy) to the beginning of your practice, or do only Restorative Yoga until you feel better.

APPENDIX B
Prop Resource Guide

Props support our practice. Most importantly, they minimize muscular tension or contraction, and this helps the body and nervous system to relax. For the practices in this book, you will need a bolster or cushion, several blankets, two blocks, and an eye pillow. You can choose to purchase props designed specifically for your yoga practice, but it's not necessary that you do so. *Chances are you already have in your home most of what you need for the practice.*

Whether you purchase props or use what you already have, remember that props are not performance-based. They support you, create comfort, and maximize relaxation so you can get the most

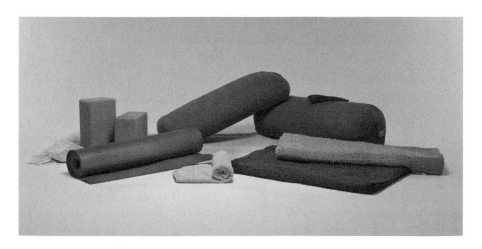

out of your practice. Instead of feeling that you need to "get it right," simply allow yourself to observe your body and mind. Use your growing awareness to determine whether you need more support or less, or whether further adjustments should be made. This will help you get the most out of your practice. This section explores the props you'll need—both purchased and in-home versions—and gives you instructions on how to use them.

YOGA OR EXERCISE MAT

In an active yoga practice, mats matter. Practitioners can spend hours researching mat stickiness (to avoid slipping), thickness, and environmental friendliness. In your Restorative Yoga practice, however, you don't need a designer mat. You just need a layer of support to cushion the floor underneath you. You can choose any sort of sticky mat, or use a mat you already have. The three most important elements of a good mat are support, comfort, and size. You'll use your mat to support you so that the surface you're lying on doesn't feel too hard on the back or front of your body. For this reason, you can use any supportive exercise mat you wish; it can be thin, like a traditional yoga mat, or puffy, like some exercise mats.

Substitutions

If you don't have a mat, you can practice on a rug in your home (the thicker the better), or on a padded surface of any kind. You can even use a blanket. Just make sure, when you practice, that the mat or rug you choose is larger than your body so that no part of your body, especially your head, hangs off the edge.

BOLSTERS

A bolster is a round, oblong cushion like a couch cushion. It supports the length of your spine, torso, and head in forward-bending postures and goes underneath the back of your legs in back-bending postures. Bolsters are stuffed with foam or environmentally friendly material such as kapok. A round bolster typically measures 27 inches long and 9 inches wide. Its length and height make it ideal for forward-bending (face-down) postures such as Child's Pose and Reclining Twist. Rectangular bolsters measure 6 inches high, 12 inches wide, and 24 inches long. However, rectangular bolsters may not have the thickness necessary to support you in Child's Pose or Reclining Twist. If you purchase a bolster, choose one round bolster, one round and one rectangular, or two rectangular ones.

Substitutions
If you don't have a bolster, good alternatives include a couch cushion, a comforter, or several thick blankets (stacked several times). If possible, your makeshift comforter-bolster or blanket-bolster should approximate the dimensions outlined above for round bolsters. Lie on your makeshift bolster; if it's puffy and you sink to the floor, you can increase its height.

BLANKETS

Yoga blankets, often called "Mexican blankets," are typically made of cotton or wool. Their dimensions are approximately 60 inches by 80 inches, and they weigh about 3 pounds. You will need three or more blankets for your Restorative Yoga practice. When you bend forward, you'll use the blankets lengthwise on top of the bolster to support your torso (as in Child's Pose and Reclining Twist). In Child's Pose, you may also roll part of a blanket under your ankles, place a folded blanket behind your knees, or put a blanket roll under your feet. In Reclining Twist, you will use a blanket folded four times between your shins to support your hips in an open, relaxed position. You may also use a blanket folded four times to support your forearm in forward-bending restorative poses such as Child's Pose and Reclining Twist.

In back-bending (face-up) restorative poses, you'll place one or two blankets lengthwise underneath you to support your spine. You may also put a folded blanket widthwise under the back of your head for neck support. If you practice Legs-up-the-Wall Pose, you will place 1–2 folded, stacked blankets under your hips.

Substitutions
If you wish, you can make do with comforters or blankets that you already have in your home. It's best if they match the thickness and dimension of yoga blankets.

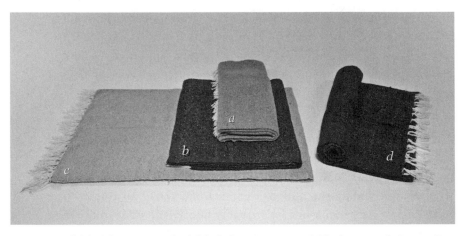

a. folded four times, b. folded three times, c. folded twice, d. foot roll

Blanket-Folding Directions

To learn the different ways you'll fold your blankets during your Restorative Yoga practice, see the instructions below and the accompanying illustration above.

FOLDED FOUR TIMES

(For use under the buttocks in Legs up the Wall Pose between the shins in Reclining Twist and Side Lying Pose, as forearm support in Child's Pose and Reclining Twist, as head support for hyperextended neck, support for behind the knees in Child's Pose, and as additional height on top of bolster for height in Child's Pose)

1. Start with your blanket completely unfolded. Then, fold it in half lengthwise, so that it makes a very long rectangle.
2. Fold in half again widthwise, so you cut the length by half.
3. Fold it one more time widthwise, so you cut the length in half a second time.
4. Fold it one more time widthwise, so you cut the length in half a third time.

FOLDED THREE TIMES

(For head support)

1. Start with your blanket completely unfolded. Then, fold it in half lengthwise, so that it makes a very long rectangle.
2. Fold in half again widthwise, so you cut the length by half.

3. Fold it one more time widthwise, so you cut the length in half a second time.

FOLDED THREE TIMES, I.E. LONG AND THIN (not shown)
(For use in Face-Down Relaxation Pose)
1. Start with your blanket completely unfolded. Then fold the blanket in half lengthwise (so you cut the width in half).
2. Fold the blanket once again lengthwise (so you cut the width in half a second time).
3. Fold once again lengthwise (so you cut the width in half a third time).

Note: If you are very tall, begin by folding lengthwise once. Then, fold widthwise. Then, fold in thirds lengthwise.

FOLDED TWICE
(For use in Inversion Pose, Relaxation Pose, and also in Side Lying Pose)
1. Start with your blanket completely unfolded. Then fold the blanket in half lengthwise (so you cut the width in half).
2. Fold once widthwise, so you make the blanket half as long as before.
3. In Supported Inversion Pose, you may choose to stack two twice-folded blankets, one on top of the other.

FOOT ROLL
(For the feet in Child's Pose)
1. Start with your blanket completely unfolded. Then fold the blanket in half lengthwise (so you cut the width in half).
2. Fold once widthwise, so you make the blanket half as long as before.
3. Starting with the rounded (uniform) edge, begin to roll the edge tightly so that it makes a large roll. Keep the roll as even as possible, so that it's the same height under each foot.

FOUR-INCH FOLD (not shown)
(For use in Gentle Backbend)
1. Start with your blanket completely unfolded. Then fold the blanket in half lengthwise (so you cut the width in half).
2. Fold the blanket widthwise (so you cut the length in half).
3. Fold the rounded edge over so that you have a 4-inch fold.

BLOCKS

Two yoga blocks will be helpful for your practice. Yoga blocks are typically 4 inches high, 6 inches wide, and 9 inches long. It is best if they are made out of foam rather than wood, as wood can be too hard. You will use the blocks in Butterfly Pose to support your thighs in an open position.

Substitutions

Thick pillows or small couch cushions are good substitutes for yoga blocks. Just make sure that they are not too low. When your legs are bent with your knees out to the side in a butterfly position, the pillows or cushions you use should keep your inner thighs from overstretching. If you feel your inner thigh muscles begin to strain or contract in Butterfly Pose, raise the height of the pillows or cushions you are using, or draw them closer in to your hips.

EYE PILLOWS

An eye pillow is a small pillow filled with flaxseeds and occasionally herbs, such as lavender. It fits over your eyes or can be placed on your forehead, just above your browbone. Eye pillows help to shut out the light and reduce sensory stimulation. The slight pressure on your eyeballs also helps to relax your eyes and also stimulates the relaxation response. Eye pillows can be especially helpful for people who struggle with insomnia.

Substitutions

If you don't have an eye pillow, you can fill a clean sock with rice. Your homemade eye pillow should weigh about 4–7 ounces. If you don't want weight on your eyes, you can fold a hand towel (see folding instructions below) and place it over your eyes. Although a towel weighs very little and won't have the same effect as a homemade eye pillow, it will still help shut out the light and reduce sensory stimulation so that your nervous system can balance.

HAND TOWEL OR DISH TOWEL

Typically, hand towels and dish towels are similar in size. They measure anywhere from 14 inches by 21 inches, to 21 inches by 28 inches. They are ideal for covering your eyes. To create an eye cover, fold your hand towel or dish towel lengthwise, in thirds, to make a long, thick 4-inch-wide fold that tucks around most of your head.

Your towels can also serve as support under your shoulders in Child's Pose (when you are forward bending). You may also choose to use them under the shoulders in Relaxation Pose and other back-bending poses, if your body requires that additional support. For "shoulder pads," or shoulder support, first fold your towel in half lengthwise, so you cut the width of the towel in half. Then, fold widthwise, so you cut the length in half. You will either use this level, or you can fold once again widthwise, thereby cutting the length in half a second time. Your towel will now be folded to make a thick square. You may use this thickness, or half of this thickness under each shoulder blade if your body would like less support.

You can also use your towel as a neck roll to provide support directly under your cervical spine. This is an alternative to using a folded blanket. You can also try both a blanket and a neck roll to see which feels more comfortable. To make a neck roll, fold your towel in half lengthwise to make a long, thin strip. Then roll it up widthwise, tightly and smoothly. Try different heights under your neck; you might choose a small neck roll, which will cause most of the towel to trail out behind your head. Or you may want a thicker neck roll, which requires that you use most of the towel or even add part of a second one. Check in with your head and neck to see which thickness works best for you. Your neck is a delicate area, so support is important. Some clues that your neck is strained and needs a towel roll are: hyperextension of your head and neck (which means your head will tilt back), strain in your throat, and difficulty breathing. Place your hands gently on your throat to ensure that your throat is relaxed. You'll be able to feel, using your hands, whether your throat is strained or at ease.

WEIGHTING YOUR POSES

In each of the four practices, you'll have the option to "weight" your poses. The added weight on top of your body can feel grounding and calming if you have anxiety and can also feel comforting and supportive if you have depression. Weighting a pose involves placing an extra bolster, blanket, pillow, or meditation cushion (sometimes called a *zafu*), on top of your abdomen or lengthwise (if you are using a long bolster for weighting) down your body. If your body likes the extra weight and feels comfortable, continue weighting your poses. If the weight feels oppressive, just remove it. When weighting a pose, use only soft weight and avoid placing blocks, books, bricks, or anything hard on top of your body.

NOTES

PREFACE

1. Throughout this book, I've included anecdotes from students and clients I've worked with over the years. Some have given me permission to use their names; others have asked me to change them. In some cases, I've used composite anecdotes (combinations of two or more stories) to protect clients' identities. I've chosen each story for its ability to represent the kinds of suffering and improvement my clients have experienced.

CHAPTER ONE: UNDERSTANDING ANXIETY AND DEPRESSION

1. J. J. Daubenmier, "The Relationship of Yoga, Body Awareness, and Body Responsiveness to Self-Objectification and Disordered Eating," *Psychology of Women Quarterly* 29, no. 2 (June 2005), 207–19.
2. V. E. Wilson and E. Peper, "The Effects of Upright and Slumped Postures on the Recall of Positive and Negative Thoughts," *Applied Psychophysiology and Biofeedback* 29, no. 3 (September 2004), 189–95.
3. C. C. Streeter, J. E. Jensen, R. M. Perlmutter, H. J. Cabral, H. Tian, D. B. Terhune, D. A. Ciraulo, and P. F. Renshaw, "Yoga Asana Sessions Increase Brain GABA Levels: A Pilot Study," *Journal of Alternative and Complementary Medicine* 13, no. 4 (May 2007), 419–26.
4. R. P. Brown, P. L. Gerbarg, "Yoga Breathing, Meditation, and Longevity," *Annals of the New York Academy of Sciences*, 1172 (August 2009), 54–62.

CHAPTER TWO: WHAT GETS IN THE WAY OF CHANGE

1. David Sipress, *New Yorker* (August 20, 2007).

CHAPTER THREE: HOW TRUE HEALING HAPPENS

1. The Zone of Proximal Development was initially developed by Lev Vygotsky, a psychologist and social learning theorist. It refers to the gap between what someone has learned and what they are able to master with assistance.

CHAPTER FOUR: FIVE WAYS TO TRANSFORM YOUR EMOTIONAL PATTERNS

1. "Yoga in America," 2008 market study, *Yoga Journal*, www.yogajournal.com/advertise/press_releases/10.
2. C. C. Streeter, J. E. Jensen, R. M. Perlmutter, H. J. Cabral, H. Tian, D. B. Terhune, D. A. Ciraulo, and P. F. Renshaw, "Yoga Asana Sessions Increase Brain GABA Levels: A Pilot Study," *Journal of Alternative and Complementary Medicine* 13, no. 4 (May 2007), 419–26.
3. Roger Cole, "Relaxation: Physiology and Practice" (April 16, 2003). Unpublished.
4. Sutra 1.2, the second of the Yoga Sutras, states that yoga is the stilling of the changing states of the mind. Bryant, Edwin F. *The Yoga Sutras of Patanjali* (New York: North Point Press, 2009).